The Power of Maca

PERUVIAN SUPERFOOD

LORRIE INGRAM B.H.SC(HONS), RHN, RNCP

ActNatural Corporation
5948 3rd Line RR#1
Hillsburgh, ON
N0B 1Z0

ISBN: 978-0-9867247-0-1

Cover and Book Design: BbM Graphics
Copy Editing: Bruce W. Cole, Cole Communications
Photo courtesy of Kim Rogers

Disclaimer:
While all care is taken with the accuracy of the facts and procedures in this book,
the author accepts neither liability nor responsibility to any person with respect to
loss, injury or damage caused, or alleged to be caused directly or indirectly, by the
information contained in this book.

The purpose of this book is to educate and inform. For medical advice you should
seek the individual, personal advice and services of a medical professional.

Printed in Canada

contents

Dedication

I dedicate this book to my best friend, my loving husband Nick. You have always given me unconditional love and support. You have always believed in me and your encouraging words are so well timed and greatly appreciated.

I love you more each day.

Special Thanks

I would like to thank Deane Parkes for believing in me and seeing the vision for this book before I did. Thank you so much for this wonderful opportunity. It has been such a fabulous experience.

I would like to thank my parents, Rodger and Cathy, for teaching me the sky is the limit. Your ongoing support has always been my foundation. And Mom – thank you for all your suggestions and feedback. They are always appreciated.

Last, but surely not least, I want to thank my dear friend Pip. Your excitement and enthusiasm about this project has been fabulous. Your daily encouraging messages along with your positive, upbeat energy has been so greatly appreciated. You are truly a wonderful friend and I thank you for your continual support.

Preface

I was sixteen years old when I became interested in holistic health. It first began with incorporating exercise into my life. I then discovered a whole foods lifestyle and began eating foods that were very different than my family. This "phase" turned into a true passion for the healing benefits of food.

As the years passed, my interest in the holistic field grew and I completely adopted this way of living. I was fascinated that you could improve your health with the use of food and that so many fabulous foods had so much healing power.

While beginning my nutritional consulting practice, I was presented with the opportunity to purchase my local health food store. Feeling that nutritional supplements and holistic nutrition were complimentary of each other, I jumped at this chance and took ownership. With my interest in rebalancing the body with whole foods and my passion for helping others, I knew this was going to be a great fit!

I did not understand at the time how purchasing a health food store would so greatly enrich my life. I wake up each morning and go to a job that I love. I still sometimes walk into the store early in the morning, with the lights still off and I stand in awe. This is MY health food store and I get to help people every day. I have the best job ever!

Being in both worlds of holistic nutrition and nutritional supplements, I have the best combination of tools to greatly assist individuals with their health. One of my goals at my health food store is to provide the most nutrient-rich supplements to my customers and clients. This is how I discovered Maca!

I myself was struggling with unbalanced hormones and was determined that I wanted to correct the imbalance MY way, with whole foods and nutritional supplements. As a result, I began my journey with Maca. I have been using Maca since 2005 and I am confident that I can attribute my balanced health to the use of this incredible superfood.

As you read through this book, you will very quickly come to understand why this superfood and nutritional supplement is one of my favourites! Maca has so many healing benefits and I receive positive feedback from my clients/customers about how Maca has improved their life! I now invite you to find out how Maca can enrich yours…

Introduction

i have the joy of going to work each day to assist individuals with improving their health. I am absolutely thrilled to be part of their health journey when choosing natural health solutions to either improve or enhance their health and well being.

I do not believe that individuals need to live in poor health, with negative symptoms or side effects. With the use of holistic nutrition and sensible supplementation, I strongly believe there is a way to provide balance to one's body – physically, mentally and emotionally.

When an individual suffers with a negative symptom, it is the body's way of telling us that there is an imbalance, the body is suffering with a nutrient deficiency. Our body is not lacking synthetic drugs such as tylenol or aspirin. In fact, the body is lacking a specific nutrient that is creating this imbalance. As a result, this imbalance has now become a symptom.

A dear friend of mine always makes this statement in her presentations when she speaks on health. I think it is very much to the point and I want to share it with you. "If you do not take the time to care for your health now, then you better make time to be sick later."

Now, I have to ask you…do you want to feel well, live symptom- free, and start each day with energy and enthusiasm? If you are interested in improving your health and living an optimal life, then I would like to introduce you to the incredible superfood MACA!

I am very excited to share with you this collaboration of information on Maca and all of its wonderful healing benefits. This incredible superfood is ideal for athletes, busy moms, stressed-out executives and hormonally imbalanced individuals. This nutrient-rich superfood can assist with energy, brain health, menopause, libido, improve sleep and much more…you must read on to find out.

The information provided to you in this book is based on research, success with clients and customers and my personal belief of this incredibly healing food. Maca has improved the health of many individuals and I am very excited to introduce you to the world of Maca!

So let's get started!

What is Maca?

Maca is a SUPERFOOD that belongs to the cruciferous vegetable family. It is grown in harsh weather conditions on mountain tops in Peru.

Maca is scientifically known as *Lepidium Meyenii Walp* and more commonly known as any of the following; maca, maka, maino, ayak, chichita, ayak willku, or Peruvian ginseng.

Maca has a very long history of being an outstanding food source, known to provide strength, as well as increase libido and stamina within individuals.

In the time of the Incas, Maca was fed to the men going to battle to provide them with stamina and strength. This was a food that was considered to be superior and at one time restricted for use only by royalty.

In the ancient times, Maca was cooked whole in pits, layered with coals of charred earth and roots. This was called "huatia" (medicine-plants.com). Maca was also prepared by boiling, mashing and rolling the root vegetable into balls and cooking it in clay pot lined with straw. This creation was referred to as "atunca."

Maca is very versatile and can be used in many different ways. Maca's bitter butterscotch flavour is used in both sweet and savoury dishes. In Canada, we are familiar with Maca as a nutritional supplement and Canadians use Maca as a liquid tonic, in capsule form and even as a powder which can be added to smoothies and various recipes. (see Appendix for recipes with Maca powder).

Maca is often described as a root that is comparable to a turnip or a radish. This small vegetable contains a very impressive nutrient content. Maca is nutritionally made up of the following nutrients: amino acids, (alanine, arginine, aspartic acid, glutamic acid, glycine, histidine, OH-proline, isoleucine, leucine, lysine, methionine, phenylalanine, proline, sarcosine, serine, threonine, tyronsine and valine), minerals, (calcium, copper, iron, magnesium, phosporus, potassium, boron, selenium, manganese, sodium, and zinc), sterols (brassicasterol, erogosterol, ergostadienol, campesterol, sitosterol and stigmasterol), and 20 fatty acids (laric, myristic, palmitic, palmitoleic, linoleic, arachidic, steric, behanic, nervonic, ligoceric, tridecanoic, 7tridecanoic, perntandecanoic, 7-pentadecanoic, heptadecanoic, 9-heptadecanoic, nonadecanoic, 11-nonadecanoic and 15-eisosenoic). Maca also includes vitamins (A, B1, B2, B3, B12, C, D and E), along with saponins, tannins, carbohydrates, protein and benzyl isothiocyanate, p-methoxbenzyl isothiiocyanate and l-ecdysone.

In a more comprehensible format, the vegetable Maca is made up of 10.4 per cent water, 10.2 per cent proteins, 2.2 per cent lipids, 59.0 per cent hydrolysable carbohydrates, 8.5 per cent whole fibre and 4.9 per cent ash. *(Source: D.Deni,G.Migliuolo, L. Rastrelli, P.Saturmino, O. Schettino, "Chemical Composition of Lepidium meyenii" in Food Chemistry 49, USA 1994, and Garro, Virginia, Macro micro elemements de la maca, mimeo, Lima, 1999).*

This incredible list of nutrients is what makes Maca one of the most powerful medicinal foods on earth!

Maca is grown in the spectacular country of Peru, 4,000 metres above sea level. This wonderful food is grown exclusively on top of the mountains where the average temperature is 4 degrees celcius. The fields experience frequent frosts and extreme winds in the evenings and the opposite weather conditions during the day, a scorching, suffocating heat, which seems perfect for growing Maca. The soil in which Maca grows is very acidic and for any other plant or food, this environment would be less than ideal growing conditions. Maca is a superfood that is loaded with rich nutrients that are bioavailable to the body and work synergistically, to provide a whole food that gives balance to the human body in many incredible ways.

2

The Process of Growing Maca

Maca is grown by the people of Peru bi-annually. This process is very important to the proper growth of the Maca vegetable and therefore the process is carried out with great care and precision by the people of Peru.

The preparation of the fields begins in the months of March and April.

The fields need to be cleared of any overgrowth or stones in order to turn over the soil. The soil is then fertilized with sheep or Llama manure.

Sowing time (planting) begins in the months of September through to November. The seeds are mixed first; the botany seed is then mixed with the soil to create a better distribution. The covering of the seed is carried out with branches or by raking superficially to ensure the appropriate depth for planting.

Approximately eight to ten months from sowing, it is time to carefully harvest the Maca. The roots of the Maca should not wither and it is necessary to try to gather all of them while harvesting this vegetable.

Traditionally, Maca is hand-picked and dried naturally in the sun. The drying process then continues in the shade in a structure much like a garden shed for approximately two months.

Once the Maca is adequately dried, it is then stored often in a "drying barn" where it is kept for many months. If Maca is stored properly, it can remain there for several months without any deterioration. To determine if the Maca has been dried to high standards, bite strongly into the dried Maca; if it has been dried properly, there should not be an imprint of your teeth. (Hilgan Enterprises Inc).

Maca is a tuberous vegetable, meaning that it is designed to absorb and store nutrients. When Maca is planted, all the nutrients within the soil are absorbed into this amazing root vegetable. This is why the nutrient profile for Maca is so rich; every vitamin, mineral, amino acid and nutrient that is found in the soil in which Maca is planted absorbs into the vegetable itself. The thought of this is both incredible and fascinating at the same time. Because Maca extracts all the nutrients from the soil it is planted in, the land where Maca grows needs to rest for three to five years between crops. This rest allows the soil to replenish and restore the vitamins and minerals that are withdrawn in the process of growing Maca.

Maca as a Root Vegetable

Maca belongs to the cruciferous/brassicaceae family or more commonly known as the cabbage or mustard family. Foods belonging to the cruciferous family are widely considered to be healthy foods as they naturally contain high levels of vitamins and multiple nutrients with anti-cancer properties (Wikepedia, May 5, 2010).

Many of us are aware of the sharp taste of cabbage and mustard greens. Maca shares this sharp taste and is one of the reasons it is such a powerful superfood. This sharp taste is produced by an amino acid that is found in Maca called glucosinolates. Glucosinolates is an organic compound that contains sulfur, nitrogen, glucose and an amino acid. Glucosinolates are found in maca, mustard, broccoli, radish, cabbage, horseradish, brussel sprouts, kale, cauliflower and turnip. Glusosinolates are similar to an antioxidant, containing wonderful healing properties. Foods that contain glucosinolates are often recommended by natural health practitioners to increase an individual's immune system and boost energy. As well, it is used as a prevention for many different forms of cancer and inflammatory health conditions. "Epidemiological studies have consistently reported a reduction in the incidence of chronic disease such as cancer and myocardial infarction through the consumption of one or more portions of cruciferous vegetables per week" (www.ifr.ac.uk/info/science/naturalproducts/glucosinolates.htm).

The Colours of Maca!

According to a study by the *Journal of the Science of Food and Agriculture*, yellow Maca (often referred to as gold Maca) and the violet

Maca or black Maca were found to be rich in glucosinolates. In the same journal, it was noted various colours of Maca (ranging from white to yellow to red to purple to black) are believed to each contain a different biological effect. The variation of each colour is believed to have a slight difference in nutrient content. Through research, it appears that the lighter Maca root contains a less potent nutrient content. The white and yellow Maca is less nutrient rich than the red, purple and black Maca. All types of Maca provide many healing benefits. However, the black Maca appears to be superior to the rest. The black Maca contains a higher potency of the many rich nutrients that provide Maca with its incredible healing properties.

Maca as a Food

In Peru where Maca is grown, it is consumed as a food. The people of Peru use Maca in soups, stews, boiled and roasted. It is also used fresh or ground. Maca is often found in flour mixtures, breads, cakes and cookies. It is even consumed daily in beverages such as milk and water, and can be prepared hot or cold. The Maca leaves are even brewed for a daily cup of tea. Maca is also used as a social tonic in alcoholic beverages. When prepared, Maca has a sweet taste, almost a butterscotch-like flavour. Maca is consumed by individuals of all ages and is used daily in meals and beverages in its native country of Peru.

Maca is still fairly new to Canada, but with its many healing benefits, it is rapidly gaining in popularity. As Canadians become more aware of Maca's wonderful healing benefits, this superfood is gaining recognition as an incredible nutrient-rich supplement. Unfortunately, due to the unique growing conditions required to cultivate Maca, it is not possible to grow Maca here in Canada. In Canada, Maca is consumed in the forms of liquid, powder and capsule. When using powdered Maca, this fabulous nutritional supplement can be added to recipes and it can be used in prepared food. (Refer to the Appendix for recipes that include Maca powder).

Choosing Maca as a Nutritional Supplement

When choosing a nutritional supplement form of Maca, it is very important that you choose a product that has good quality control, and has undergone the gelatinization process. Gelatinized Maca contains the highest potency of the active ingredients of Maca and is optimal for absorption, which therefore produces a better product with superior results.

With all this in mind, I recommend the following product lines: **MacaPunch XP Platinum** liquid and **Brad King's Ultimate Maca Energy** in powder and capsules. All three of these nutritional supplements have great quality control, provide superior results and have undergone the gelatinization process.

Gelatinization requires an extrusion process that removes the starch from the root, leaving a more concentrated powder that is easier to digest. (MacaPunch Gelatinization Process – Hilgan Enterprises Inc). Gelatinization is a process which eliminates the components of the vegetable that are not easily absorbed by the human body. The most valuable and concentrated nutrients remain and will be optimally absorbed into the body creating positive health benefits. This process makes the **MacaPunch** line and Brad King's **Ultimate Maca Energy** different than many other brands on the market. The removal of the starch and fibre in the Maca allows for a more optimal absorption of these rich nutritional supplements.

The Gelatinization process of Maca is necessary, as raw Maca contains hydrocynanic acid, a poisonous element naturally found in raw Maca. The gelatinization process guarantees the absence of hydrocynanic acid in the Maca when used in supplement form. In addition, the absorption rate and the results an individual notices from taking Maca will be inferior if the Maca is not gelatinized. In essence, the quality will be different. (Hilgan Enterprises Inc).

MacaPunch XP Platinum is a high potency liquid Maca. This product is a unique cold-pressed, gelatinized formula using certified organic black Maca. This formula is an 18-20:1 ratio, meaning that approximately 18-20 kg of Maca makes 1 litre of Maca extract.

This liquid is ideal for an individual who requires high doses of Maca. Liquid nutritional supplements are ideal and the best way to absorb nutrients. With liquid supplementation, you are more likely to achieve your health goals more quickly.

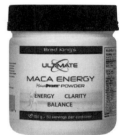

Ultimate Maca Energy powder is another form in which you can use Maca. This concentrated certified organic powder includes various colours of Maca and is easily digested and absorbed. The concentration ratio of this product is 4-6:1, meaning approximately 4-6 kg of Maca makes 1 kg of gelatinized Maca powder. The powder form of Maca is great for individuals who want to add Maca to their foods, such as shakes, smoothies, yogourt, muffins, scones and soups. In the Appendix, you will find several recipes in which Maca has been added. The powder is a great way to increase the nutrient content of some of your favourite foods and balance your system all at the same time.

The final product (which is quite popular) is Brad King's **Ultimate Maca Energy capsules**. These capsules are made with 100 per cent fair trade certified organic gelatinized Maca powder. Each capsule contains 750 mg of Maca, creating a ratio of 6:1 per capsule, meaning 6 kg of fresh Maca makes 1 kg of gelatinized Maca powder which is then put into a capsule.

The benefit to taking the Brad King's **Ultimate Maca Energy capsules** is that they are easy and convenient to use. If you are a person always on the go, or someone who travels frequently, they are great to just carry in your purse or travel bag. Also, if you are not fussy about taking liquids such as the **MacaPunch XP Platinum** and you are not interested in adding the **Ultimate Maca Energy powder** to your foods, then you are still able to benefit from the wonderful healing properties of Maca by using Brad King's **Ultimate Maca Energy capsules**.

All of the **MacaPunch** products are 100 per cent pure and naturally certified organic Maca roots. The **MacaPunch liquid** and Brad King's

Ultimate Maca Energy in powder and capsules are manufactured under strict production standards and use high quality control. All these products are made with selected dry roots, mainly the darker roots (black and red-purple Maca) and follow unique production methods. The process is an exclusive cold gelatinization process that removes the starch from the Maca root and provides the maximum bioavailability of nutrients. All **MacaPunch** products are preservative-free, do not contain fillers and are a completely natural product line, free of dangerous chemical substances. MacaPunch is one of the very few companies that bring to the world organically produced Gelatinized Maca. (MacaPunch – Hilgan Enterprises Inc).

7

Maca Options

When referring to nutritional supplementation and health, it is important to know that taking a supplement in liquid or powder form is always most ideal. When you consume a liquid form of food (such as soup or smoothie), a liquid nutritional supplement or a beverage, it is more beneficial to your digestive system and you will absorb more of the nutrients. Liquids and powders are the best vehicle for nutrients to be absorbed and less work for your digestive system to break down.

Everything that you consume (food, beverage, nutritional supplements) must go through the digestive system and be broken down by the digestive enzymes that are produced in your stomach. Once food has gone through your digestive system and is properly absorbed, that is when you feel the benefits of what you have eaten in terms of energy and well-being.

If you suffer from digestive issues such as indigestion, bloating or gas, I would absolutely recommend that you choose the liquid or powder form of any nutritional supplement, including Maca. **MacaPunch XP Platinum** liquid or **Ultimate Maca Energy powder** would be ideal for a compromised digestive system. These two forms of Maca are easily digested and your body will be able to efficiently absorb the nutrients from this fabulous superfood.

If you are choosing your Maca supplement based on convenience and ease, then Brad King's **Ultimate Maca Energy capsules** are ideal for you. These capsules are easy to use, and if you decide that you want to try the powder, just open a few capsules and put them into your morning smoothie.

Once you begin using Maca, you can switch between the various forms that are offered. At times, you may find the capsules are more convenient for you and then other times, you might find that you are suffering with some digestive issues or require a more potent dose and therefore, the liquid is a better option. To maintain your results with Maca, just be sure you consume the same dose whether you are taking liquid, powder or capsules.

Use and Dosage of Maca

The way in which you consume Maca is individual. The most important aspect of adding Maca to your health regime is to be consistent in taking adequate amounts for the health condition you are trying to rebalance. As a general suggestion, 3000 to 5000 mg of Maca per day is a standard dose. If you are using liquid, I would recommend one teaspoon, three times a day as a standard dose.

When comparing the dose of **MacaPunch XP Platinum liquid** versus Brad King's **Ultimate Maca Energy powder** or **Ultimate Maca Energy capsules**, it is important to understand that the liquid is more concentrated and therefore, more potent. (**MacaPunch XP Platinum** liquid 18-20:1 versus Brad King's **Ultimate Maca Energy powder** or **Ultimate Maca Energy capsules** 6:1).

Essentially, the liquid is three times stronger than the capsule or powder form. So to make it easier to understand, one teaspoon of **MacaPunch XP Platinum** liquid is approximately equivalent to three teaspoons of **Ultimate Maca Energy powder** or three capsules of **Ultimate Maca Energy**.

In terms of dosage, I would recommend that you consume Maca in divided doses. For example, if you are taking six **Ultimate Maca**

Energy capsules per day, I would recommend that you take two capsules at each breakfast, lunch and dinner. I would not suggest that you consume the full dose of six capsules at once. I believe the body is better able to absorb nutrients when provided in small doses, frequently throughout the day. To provide you with a comparison, health experts know that it is more beneficial to our digestion, as well as our energy levels if we consume three to five small meals per day, as opposed to one large meal. One large meal per day is very difficult in terms of the body breaking down such a large amount of food at one time and absorbing the nutrients. As well, it is more beneficial and more effective to replenish our bodies with food frequently to maintain optimal energy levels. Replenishing the body with nutritional supplements continuously throughout the day will allow your body to absorb the maximum amount of nutrients from each supplement. Consuming Maca in divided doses will allow you to experience the many benefits that Maca provides throughout your whole day.

Maca is a superfood consumed in supplement form to provide individuals that do not live in Peru the opportunity to experience the wonderful healing effects that Maca has to offer. Maca is a very safe food/nutritional supplement and you can achieve great healing benefits from adding this superfood to your life. Both men and women experience improved health with the use of Maca. One of the most exciting aspects of Maca is that there are not any known side effects of using this fabulous superfood. Maca is safe and effective for individuals of all ages.

This wonderful superfood is full of rich nutrients that will assist in bringing your body back into balance. Maca is a nutrient-packed nutritional supplement, not a magic potion. When using Maca, keep in mind that the body is a magnificent machine and can heal itself with the use of the necessary nutrients. However, the system that you are correcting did not come out of balance as a result of one day of poor lifestyle or food choices. So when using Maca, be consistent and understand that the results may not be instant for everyone. Some individuals have reported results within a couple days to a week, while with others, it has taken up to six weeks to see improvements in their health. With any hormonal regime, it is very standard to use a nutritional supplement consistently for six weeks before significant results are noticed. Keep in mind repairing a nutrient-deficient body requires time.

In my five years of recommending Maca, I can confidently report that the majority of my clients noticed positive results sooner than the six week time frame. Often, increase in energy and mental clarity are the first improvements they report – even when those were not the initial health complaint. My clients who take their nutritional supplements consistently throughout the day achieve balance within their systems more quickly and report improvement of symptoms in a shorter period of time.

As you develop a better quality of life – including a balanced hormonal system and a true sense of wellness – Maca is the type of nutrient that when you start taking it, you will notice when you have missed it.

As you read further in this book, you will find that as I discuss various health concerns, I have provided a specific protocol with the recommended dosages for Maca in both liquid and capsule form. You will notice that the dosage varies depending on the condition that is being discussed. I have developed these protocols from research and through working with my clients to find the therapeutic dose of Maca required to provide the most effective results for the specific health concern being examined.

With Maca's incredible nutritional profile, the multiple options for consuming Maca and the quality of the product produced, it is a wonder that every individual is not already taking this fabulous superfood! With the various ailments that many of us struggle with every day, it is time to examine how Maca can help you to experience a greater quality of life!

Healing Benefits of Maca!

Maca is a nutrient that is beneficial for both males and females. For women, Maca can enhance libido, increase aphrodisiac activity, increase energy, stamina and endurance, increase sexual stimulation, assist to overcome depression and chronic fatigue, improve the immune system, increase general well-being, help fight menopausal symptoms, decrease stress and anxiety, reduce hot flashes, improve hormonal balance, and it may improve sleep patterns. Maca is an adjuvant to hormone replacement therapy (HRT) and is also known to correct menstrual irregularity and pre-menstural syndrome (PMS) issues, enhance fertility, improve concentration and state of mind.

The wonderful superfood Maca has just as much to offer to men in the way of assisting with healing and balancing their health. Maca can help men to enhance libido, increase aphrodisiac activity, increase energy, stamina and endurance, increase sperm count, mobility and formation, assist to overcome depression and chronic fatigue, improve the immune system, and increase general well-being. Maca can assist with increasing testosterone levels, and aid in erectile dysfunction. Maca assists with building muscle mass and is therefore a safe and effective alternative to steroids.

Maca is also known to increase dehydroepiandrosterone (DHEA) in most males and females. Maca is a potent antioxidant that fights aging and provides cellular protection. And last, but most definitely not least, Maca is known to provide significant rebuilding of bone density in individuals with osteoporosis.

BENEFITS FOR MEN	BENEFITS FOR WOMEN
1. Maca increases aphrodisiac activity and enhances libido.	
2. Increases energy, stamina and endurance: Improves athletic performance	
3. Improvement of male potency.	**3.** It increases sexual stimulation
4. Helps to overcome depression and chronic fatigue.	
5. Improves immune system: found to produce a "general sense of well-being"	
6. Increases DHEA in most males and females.	**6.** Helps fight menopause symptoms.
7. Maca decreases stress, anxiety and helps their treatment.	
8. Increase sperm count, mobility and formation	**8.** Reduces hot flashes
9. Hormone balancing and may improve sleep patterns	
10. Increased testosterone levels.	**10.** Adjuvant to hormone replacement therapy (HTR).
11. Assists with erectile dysfunction.	**11.** Corrects menstrual irregularity/ PMS Issues
12. Enhances Fertility	
13. Helps fight acne and related skin problems resulted from hormonal imbalances.	
14. Better concentration, clear thinking and state of mind	
15. Potent anti aging, antioxidant free radicals scavenger and provides cellular protection	
16. Alternative steroids: helps build muscle mass	**16.** Osteoporosis: significant rebuilding bone density

WOW! What a fabulous food...are you convinced yet? After reading the list of wonderful benefits that Maca has to offer, you are likely thinking EVERYONE should be taking this wonderful superfood! And you are right!

Many of us suffer with at least one of the symptoms listed above and to know that there is a natural, nutrient rich, healthy food that you can add to your diet to improve your system and assist you in feeling great is wonderful! Maca is a phenomenal superfood that truly aids in improving overall health and wellness at any age, with any individual and in both genders.

10

Stress and Maca

In today's society, many of us are overworked, over-tired, and chronically stressed. The majority of individuals lead hectic lives, always on the go with very little time left to relax and recharge. This type of lifestyle can be viewed as exciting. However the constant chaos can create a great deal of stress within the body.

According to the Canadian Mental Health Association, Canadians in 2010 were reporting a thirty per cent increase in their stress levels compared to 2009 (www.cbc.com). Daily stress rates peaked at more than twenty-eight per cent in the working-age groups thirty-five to forty-four and forty-five to fifty-four years old. These individuals are most likely to be managing multiple roles associated with career and family responsibilities, stated the Canadian Community Health Survey from Statistics Canada.

In my consulting practice, as well as in my health food store, I speak with individuals who have fallen into the above statistic. Many are overworked, tired and juggling multiple responsibilities. These individuals are looking for a supplement that will assist them to manage their stress. They are searching for a nutritional aid that will combat stress, improve their energy and provide them with overall well being. And guess what? I have the perfect solution... Maca!

When I meet these individuals, I begin educating them on the healing benefits of Maca and each time, they are very intrigued about this fascinating superfood. A food that offers the healing benefits of reducing stress and creating a feeling of wellness is virtually unheard of. However, Maca is an adaptogen and by medical definition an adaptogen "is non-toxic to the recipient, it produces a nonspecific response in the body; an increase in the power of resistance against multiple stressors including physical, chemical or biological agents and has a normalizing influence on physiology" (Israel I. Brekham, M.D., Authority on Adaptogens).

To put it simply, an adaptogen is a substance that assists the body in dealing with stress, therefore helping the body to adapt to a stressful circumstance. An adaptogen increases the body's resistance to stress, fatigue or trauma. All adaptogens contain antioxidants but not all anti-oxidants are considered an adaptogen. Maca is rich in the antioxidants, zinc, vitamins C, D, E and plant sterols.

Adaptogens have the ability to balance endocrine hormones and boost the immune system. In addition, the nutrient-rich ingredients of adaptogens provide balance to the body and maintain optimal homeostasis.

In my practice, I have witnessed the healing benefits that individuals receive by using Maca to manage their stress. Maca acts as a balancer to help the body, assisting the individual to better deal with stress, fatigue and anxiety. With Maca being an adaptogen, this superfood is designed to work *with* the body and aid in achieving balance in an otherwise chaotic or stressful environment.

With the healing properties of the antioxidants, as well as the high levels of B vitamins and magnesium that are naturally found in Maca, this food is the perfect combination for reducing stress and physically relaxing the body. B vitamins are essential for balancing the nervous system and the endocrine/hormonal system. Magnesium is a wonderful mineral that aids in physical relaxation of the body's muscles which is often necessary in an individual that is suffering with stress. Maca contains eighteen amino acids, which are naturally found in high protein foods such as chicken, turkey, beans, fish and eggs. (Refer to Appendix B for a list of quality protein sources). The proper balance of amino acids within an individual is what dictates how the individual will feel in terms of mood. If you have the proper balance of amino acids in your diet, then you will feel more positive, upbeat and energetic. If you are lacking in amino acids, then you are more prone to feeling depressed, angry and suffer with anxiety.

(Julia Ross, The Mood Cure 2002, pg 7). This aspect is very important when we are dealing with stress. If you are lacking these very important nutrients, then even the small everyday stresses are going to overwhelm you.

One study found that the amino acid glucosinolates naturally occurring in Maca has been proven to significantly improve anti-stress activity in mice that were exposed to stress induced by electrical stimulation. (Anti- Stress Effects of two Extracts of Maca Enriched in Glucosinolates. Capcha R, Marcelo A, Rojas P, Ramos A, Aguilar JL).

It is incredible that Maca contains eighteen of the twenty-two amino acids, along with multiple antioxidants, high B vitamins and magnesium. This superfood is a nutrient-rich, anti-stress formula created by Mother Nature.

With this astounding nutritional profile, it is no wonder that Maca provides amazing results for those suffering with chronic stress, anxiety and depression. This is the ideal combination to physically calm the body, relax the mind and at the same time assist the body to build a healthy store of energy. Maca provides the perfect combination of nutrients to reorganize and recharge, along with building stamina in a highly stressed body.

Maca Protocol:

One teaspoon of **MacaPunch XP Platinum**, twice daily, or three capsules of Brad King's **Ultimate Maca Energy capsules**, twice daily.

Nutrition Tips:

▶ Focus on a whole foods lifestyle (Refer to Appendix A for a complete Introduction to a Whole Foods Lifestyle). When the body is exhausted and stressed, it is important that you ingest quality nutrients. If you are consuming packaged and processed foods, this will create more stress within your body and you will feel more agitated. The packaged and processed foods do not offer any nutritional content to support a stressed system.

▶ An abundance of fruits and vegetables (five to six servings per day, one serving is equivalent to ½ cup) to provide high antioxidant content.

▶ Quality protein (Refer to Appendix B for a list of quality protein sources)

▶ Include four to five servings of protein per day. (3oz is equivalent to one serving)

▶ A nutrient-rich diet of fruits, vegetables and protein will provide the body with the necessary ingredients to increase energy and more adequately deal with stress.

Adrenal Fatigue and Maca

In general, our lifestyles are very busy and we are always on the go! We have work, family, financial and social responsibilities and the list goes on and on. As I discussed in the previous section, stress is a common problem and Maca can assist with managing these stresses. As individuals, we have many activities crammed into an unreasonable amount of time. We are busy with multiple commitments, some of which we thoroughly enjoy and some of which we do not. Regardless of what is keeping us busy, we are always running to the next appointment or the next activity. Having a life that is constantly on the go is what creates the chronic stress in our bodies. Sometimes the stress can become so overwhelming that we reach a point of feeling burnt out. When we get to this point, the body is not able to handle any level of stress – physical, mental or emotional. Due to the high level of stress that has become chronic, the body is nutrient-deficient and does not have the necessary fuel to fight back. When stress becomes this serious, it is referred to as Adrenal Fatigue.

Adrenal Fatigue is when an individual's stress glands – known as the adrenal glands – are no longer able to cope with the level of stress that is being placed on the body, whether it be physical, mental, emotional or a combination of all three.

The purpose of the adrenal glands is to assist the body in coping with stresses and survive. (Adrenal Fatigue, Wilson, 2001, pg3). The adrenal glands are known as our stress glands and their job is to enable the body to deal with stress of any kind. "No bigger than a walnut and weighing less than a grape, each of your two adrenal glands sits like a tiny pyramid on top of a kidney" (Adrenal Fatigue, Wilson, 2001, pg3).

The adrenal glands affect the functioning of every tissue, organ and gland in the body. This gland is an extremely important part of the body's make up. The adrenal gland affects how you think and feel, as well as your response to incoming stress to your body and mind. How well your adrenal glands are functioning will dictate how your body and mind responds to stress, whether it be a small stress such as running late for an appointment or a large stress such the death of a loved one.

Unfortunately, when it comes to stress, our bodies cannot distinguish the difference between good and bad stress. The same physiological responses occur (heart palpitations, rising blood pressure, nervous energy, dilating pupils, increase in body temperature and sweating) when we experience a negative stress (loved one is sick) as compared to a positive stress (you just got married).

If you think of all the times that you have been happy (fantastic adrenal pumping excitement) to devastated sorrow, your body goes through the same physiological responses with each experience. When you have a life that is constantly on the go and you do not stop and enjoy relaxation time, your body does not have the opportunity to replenish your system. The body is in constant adrenaline pumping mode, without any time to restore balance. It is very important that we all take "down time," exercise regularly to reduce stress, have a bath at night to wind down or take a book to bed to read and relax. By including relaxing activities into our day, it provides the body a chance to rejeuvenate and rebuild our energy stores to prepare for the next day. If we do not incorporate any relaxation time in our day, then our bodies constantly stay in a hyper stress mode. When the body is functioning in a high-stressed state consistently, this creates an individual who is always feeling rushed, stressed, tired and overwhelmed. This is the process that an individual goes through when they have reached Adrenal Fatigue and unfortunately, it is more common than many of us would like to admit.

Stress is a part of everyday life and how you perceive your stress and what you do to balance your stress will dictate whether it has a positive or negative effect on your health.

Hans Selye, a Canadian physician and one of the early pioneers of modern stress theory, defined stress as; "the nonspecific response of the body to any demand, whether it is caused by, or results in, pleasant or unpleasant conditions."

Selye also identified three stages of adaptation which a person experiences during a time of stress. He called this General Adaptation Syndrome. These are the three stages that he identified as the experience an individual goes through each time they are presented with stress. The first stage is Alarm, (the immediate response to the stressful event), the second stage is Resistance/Adaptation (the body's response to long term protection-begin to adapt to the level of stress even if it is unhealthy) and the third stage is Exhaustion (the stress has been constant and the body is no longer able to cope and becomes tired).

The three defined stages are all associated with biological changes that happen within the body during the time of stress. During the three stages, the body gradually produces more "stress hormone" known as cortisol. If the stress continues for an extended period of time and becomes chronic, then the body will eventually be depleted of the required nutrients and resources to deal with the stress. The ultimate result is complete physical, emotional and mental exhaustion.

We are presented with stressors numerous times throughout the day, every day. So it is very important that the body has the required nutrients to deal with all of these stresses appropriately and effectively.

The adrenal glands produce several hormones and all the hormones are imperative for proper functioning of the endocrine, nervous and reproductive systems. The hormones secreted by the adrenal glands influence all major physiological processes that occur within the body. These hormones affect the "utilization of carbohydrates and fats, the conversion of fats and proteins into energy, the distribution of stored fat (especially around the waist and at the sides of your face), normal blood sugar regulation, and proper cardiovascular and gastrointestinal function" (Adrenal Fatigue, Wilson, 2001, pg4).

An individual that is suffering with Adrenal Fatigue could suffer any or all of the following symptoms; difficulty getting out of bed in the morning, feelings of extreme fatigue even after a full night's rest, cravings for salt or salty foods, increased effort to complete everyday tasks and lethargy. As well, this individual could suffer with decreased sex drive, decreased ability to handle stress, poor healing – taking the body longer to recover from illness, injury or trauma – and light-headedness when standing up too quickly. Symptoms such as mild depression, less enjoyment or happiness in life (activities or events previously enjoyed), increased PMS, symptoms worsen when you miss or skip meals, fuzzy thinking, brain fog, poor memory, irritablity and less tolerance than normal could all be possible indications of adrenal fatigue.

The symptoms listed above contribute to an overall feeling of unwell, being run down and having a lack of motivation. The symptoms of Adrenal Fatigue can go unnoticed because often individuals will ignore the symptoms or simply relate them to being stressed or just tired. And the truth of the matter is they are right! The individual is stressed AND tired and the organ in the body that is designed to provide you with energy to cope is now running on empty. Without supporting the adrenal gland, this very important organ, you will become chronically stressed and tired and you will not remember the last time you truly felt rested and well! When this is the way you experience your life, the symptoms of Adrenal Fatigue become your "normal." This in fact is how you function and you do not realize that you are run down, overwhelmed and exhausted. You have been living this way for so long that you cannot recognize these symptoms as unbalanced and very unhealthy.

The Adrenal Fatigue symptoms listed is your body's way of telling you that you are out of balance and require specific nutrients to replenish and restore your system. Those symptoms can be related to many different health conditions and sometimes being tired is just that, you were busy today and feel tired. However, when you are always tired and overwhelmed, even after a good night sleep, this is a chronic issue that requires attention. Now it is time for you to do your part and listen to what your body is trying to tell you.

An individual suffering with Adrenal Fatigue not only needs to adjust their lifestyle to include more relaxation and personal 'Me' time, but this individual also needs specific nutrients to feed their endocrine system, as well as the nervous system. Both of these systems are running on empty and attempting to deal with chronic stress and unfortunately failing miserably.

Remember earlier where I listed all the nutrients that naturally occur in Maca? High B vitamins, amino acids, antioxidants and magnesium – all of these nutrients are beneficial for balancing and supporting the endocrine system and the nervous system. The nutrients found in Maca will ultimately increase an individual's energy and provide balance to the body and reduce stress levels. It is amazing that Maca is loaded with all the nutrients required for an individual to recover from Adrenal Fatigue.

Magnesium is a very important mineral that is beneficial to the physical body in the way of relaxation and is necessary for an individual suffering with Adrenal Fatigue. Often with Adrenal Fatigue, the individual will feel achy all over, experience sore muscles and feel physically defeated. Naturally occurring magnesium, in Maca, will assist with relaxing the tense muscles within the body. An individual that is suffering with chronic stress will also be suffering with muscle tension throughout their body. Providing magnesium on a regular basis to the muscles will allow them to begin to relax and therefore reduce the overall physical feeling of tension within the body.

Regular consumption of nutrient-rich Maca is important to assist the body in dealing with chronic stress. Adrenal fatigue is corrected by providing the adrenal glands the necessary nutrients to build up the stores of these high functioning glands. Designing your schedule with more relaxation time will provide further assistance to maintaining healthy adrenal glands once they have been replenished.

I cannot emphasize enough how significant the necessary nutrients are to overcoming Adrenal Fatigue. A regular intake of Maca is essential along with a healthy wholesome diet. Both are critical to general health and imperative for recovering from Adrenal Fatigue.

A study was conducted on the effects that Maca has on animals experiencing stress. The results showed a significantly lower score of stress in the mice that were supplemented with Maca compared to the control group. In addition, the mice that were supplemented with Maca were found to be able to normalize themselves more quickly after being exposed to stress. Therefore, this study was successful in supporting that supplementing with Maca has anti-stress effects in an animal model. (Maca and its Anti-Stress Effect in an Animal Model in Mice. Tapia A, Lopez C, Marcelo A, Canales M, Aguilar JL. Acta Andina 1999-2000;8:31-37).

Maca Protocol:

One teaspoon of **MacaPunch XP Platinum** liquid, four times a day, or three capsules of Brad King's **Ultimate Maca Energy**, four times a day. (continue this dose for three to six months depending on the severity of the symptoms).

A maintenance dose of two teaspoons of **MacaPunch XP Platinum** liquid per day or six capsules of Brad King's **Ultimate Maca Energy** is beneficial to maintain healthy adrenal glands.

Additional Nutrient Recommendations:

Multi-Vitamin: ideally one capsule with each meal. This provides constant replenishment of nutrients. Read the label and be sure that it contains at least 50mg of each B vitamin.

B Complex 50mg: one capsule or one tablespoon, three times a day.

Nutrition Tips:

The food an individual consumes as fuel for the body is very important to improve Adrenal Fatigue. Refer to *Appendix A – Introduction to a Whole Foods Lifestyle* and begin to incorporate many of these foods into your daily diet.

Eliminate white flour products, white sugar, caffeine, alcohol and processed foods to assist your body in dealing with the high level of stress. These foods create more stress in your body. Processed and packaged foods do not offer enough quality nutrients to assist in the recovery of Adrenal Fatigue. When an individual is suffering with Adrenal Fatigue, it is necessary to eat foods that are full of nutrients such as fresh fruits, raw vegetables, quality proteins, wholesome grains and omega 3 fats. What you put into your system both in terms of nutrition and supplements is what fuels your health! High quality food and nutritional supplementation will provide a high-functioning body with great energy and an overall feeling of wellness.

Lifestyle Suggestions:

Recognizing that Adrenal Fatigue is not just a nutrient deficiency but also an unbalanced lifestyle is a very important part of the healing process. Adjusting one's lifestyle to assist with providing more balance to maintain a healthy level of stress is crucial. This includes designating quality 'Me' time where you are involved in activities that you truly enjoy and are stress relievers. This could be exercise, meditation, gardening, quiet time with a loved one or this could be more traditional relaxation, such as taking a hot bubble bath or curling up with a good book. Whatever activities you find relaxing, they need to be incorporated into your daily life. Everyone needs personal time and when you are suffering with Adrenal Fatigue.Your body is telling you loud and clear that you are not taking enough time for YOU!

Receiving good quantity and quality sleep is a major factor in recovery of Adrenal Fatigue. Often, sleeplessness is a sign of Adrenal Fatigue, so getting quality sleep is sometimes an issue. Individuals suffering with Adrenal Fatigue will often find they have trouble waking up in the morning, but get their second wind or burst of energy after 11pm in the evening. If this describes you, then it is important that you be on your way to bed between 10:00–10:30pm and try to be asleep by 11:00pm. If you stay up past 11:00pm, you will find that you have caught that second wind and you may find yourself awake until 2:00am. Staying up this late will not allow your adrenal glands to restore.

In terms of ideal times for waking up, an individual suffering with Adrenal Fatigue would greatly benefit from sleeping until 8:30-9:00am every day. I know this is not realistic for many who work in the morning, but if you can stay in bed until 9:00am on the weekends or on your days off, you will be doing your adrenal glands a favour. The benefit to staying in bed until 9:00am when you suffer from Adrenal Fatigue is that the stress hormone cortisol rapidly rises between 6:00am and 8:00am in a hormonally-balanced individual. With individuals suffering with Adrenal Fatigue, the hormone cortisol often does not rise as high and/or will drop faster than normal. (Adrenal Fatigue,Wilson, 2001, pg 124,125). Being asleep at the time of the hormone production of cortisol will improve the individual's chances of producing cortisol more efficiently and more of it, which will improve energy and vitality.

The Endocrine System and Maca

The endocrine system is the major hormonal centre of our body. This very important system includes the pituitary gland (master hormonal gland – The Boss), adrenal gland (stress gland) and the thyroid gland (metabolism).

It is imperative that all three glands within the endocrine system are communicating well for the body to function at its best.

There are many health conditions that require the endocrine system to be balanced. There are times in which the glands of the endocrine system are not communicating effectively and this is when an imbalance occurs. An imbalance within the endocrine system creates a hormonal imbalance within an individual and this can happen in both men and women. Stress and Adrenal Fatigue – which was discussed in the previous section – is one of the major health conditions that can occur with a less than optimal functioning endocrine system.

Underactive Thyroid or Hypothyroidism is another very common health condition that is a result of an imbalance within the endocrine system. Over ten million Canadians are affected with some form of thyroid imbalance or thyroid condition (Thyroid Foundation of Canada, www.thyroid.ca).

The thyroid gland secretes hormones that are responsible for the functioning of the metabolism, regulating body functions and is essential for growth and development. This small gland is located at the base of the neck and weighs only twenty grams. Thyroid disorders are found in 0.8 per cent to 5 per cent of the population and are four to seven times more common in women than men (Thyroid Foundation of Canada, www.thyroid.ca).

Very little attention is paid to the thyroid gland unless it is not secreting the thyroid hormones required for a healthy metabolism, which often leads to weight gain. Many individuals discover they have an imbalance in their thyroid because they notice weight gain without explanation and they are suffering from extreme fatigue. Additional symptoms that can indicate your thyroid gland is not secreting adequate thyroid hormones is a weak, slow heart beat, muscular weakness, sensitivity to the cold, thick puffy skin and/or dry skin, slowed mental processes, poor memory, constipation and goiter,a condition where the size of the thyroid gland itself enlarges (Thyroid Foundation of Canada, www.thyroid.ca).

The endocrine system works in synchronization and all team players need to be present and active for the system to function well as a whole. The fact that all of these glands are interconnected is the very reason that I feel that it is important to cover the thyroid gland and its relationship to the adrenals.

The thyroid gland produces two very important hormones – tetraiodo-thyronine (thyroxine or T4) and triiodothyronine (T3) – which are responsible for regulating physiological functions within the body such as metabolism, growth and development as previously mentioned. If an individual is diagnosed with the condition of an under-active thyroid, this means the thyroid gland is failing to produce the required amount of T4 hormone for optimal functioning. When someone experiences the onset of under-active thyroid, all the organs within the body go into a '"hypo-function –mode,"' basically slowing down the entire endocrine system. This results in the possibility that all the hormones that are produced by the endocrine system could slow down and affect the overall functioning of the individual.

The adrenals are a part of the endocrine system. Some medical researchers and many natural health care practitioners believe that the cortisol (stress hormone) the adrenal gland secretes provides assistance to the thyroid gland to perform its metabolic regulating activities. Consequently, an individual suffering with Adrenal Fatigue would essentially be suffering with less than optimal thyroid function as well. Putting these two conditions together, this individual will be suffering with intense fatigue, mood swings, depression, weight gain, lack of concentration and lack of motivation. These are symptoms commonly shared by both adrenal fatigue and under-active thyroid.

Dr.Gloria Chacon, a researcher and expert on Maca, suggests that with the regular use of Maca, the hormonal system can be balanced. In her research Dr. Chacon found that Maca contains alkaloids. The National Institute of Cancer defines alkaloids as "a member of a large group of chemicals that are made by plants and have nitrogen in them. Some alkaloids have been shown to work against cancer." (www.cancer.gov). Dr. Chacon suggests that the alkaloids in Maca "act on the hypothalamus-pituitary axis and the adrenals." Her research supports that taking Maca balances the master gland, the hypothalamus. With the hypothalamus balanced, this provides regulation to the other endocrine glands, including the pituitary, adrenals, ovaries, testes, thyroid and pancreas. We know that the endocrine system works synergistically, so when the master gland is balanced, this provides balance to the entire endocrine system.

In addition to Dr. Chacon's research on Maca's "balancing" properties, Maca is also an adaptogen, high in B vitamins and rich in antioxidants which contribute to the balancing of the hormonal system overall. As we know, when the system is stressed, it is crucial to provide the necessary nutrients to return the body back to balance. Maca is a great solution to balancing exhausted adrenals and a low functioning thyroid gland. It is interesting to know that each gland within the endocrine system becomes stronger, more balanced and therefore more efficient with the regular use of Maca. This incredible nutrient-rich Peruvian root vegetable has so much to offer and is one of the world's best kept secrets…until now!

Maca Protocol:

One teaspoon of **MacaPunch XP Platinum** liquid, four times daily or three capsules of Brad King's **Ultimate Maca Energy capsules**, four times daily

Nutrition Tip:

Individuals that have an underactive thyroid are often lacking the mineral iodine in their diet. Unfortunately there are not a lot of foods that contain high levels of the mineral iodine.

I recommend two to three servings per day of the following foods to enhance your intake of the iodine mineral to enhance the functioning of your thyroid: Haddock, eggs, sea kelp (available in health food stores), seaweed, and sea salt.

If you visit your local health food store, you will be able to purchase sea kelp in powder, tablet or capsule form. Adding one teaspoon of kelp to a smoothie is a great way to increase your intake of iodine. (Refer to the recipe section in the Appendix for great smoothie ideas).

Menstruation and Maca

The Endocrine system is responsible for many functions within the body. A very important function is the balance of the female reproductive system. Many women struggle with an imbalanced endocrine system from the time of her first menstrual cycle to the final days of menopause. Some of the symptoms that indicate an imbalance within the female's endocrine system are depression due to hormonal imbalance, mood swings, PMS, hot flashes and menopause. As well, heavy menstrual cycles, irregular menstrual cycles, under-active thyroid, low libido, headaches and fatigue are additional symptoms that indicate hormonal imbalance. These symptoms are letting you know that your endocrine system is not producing the required level of hormones that are necessary to create a healthy functioning body.

The great news is that these symptoms can be significantly decreased and can even be eliminated when you provide the necessary nutrients to balance the endocrine system. These symptoms are your body's way of getting your attention to tell you that your hormonal system is in need of support and nutrient replenishment.

Maca is the solution to increase your natural hormone production and provide hormonal balance.

TESTIMONIAL FROM JULIE, AGE 49

*I started using Brad King's **Ultimate Maca Energy capsules** years ago. I first started using Brad King's **Ultimate Maca Energy capsules** when I was working out three hours a day for muscle recovery. I then began to incorporate Brad King's **Ultimate Maca Energy capsules** when I was stressed, even for the day-to- day stress. Then, later in life as my PMS turned to menopause, I again turned to Brad King's **Ultimate Maca Energy capsules**. Being the mother of two daughters I have been able to see Maca work on all age groups from teenagers to middle age and I expect to continue using Maca into my later years. Maca is a savior for women! – You know, God can't be everywhere!*

Maca is a hormone balancer and a hormone regulator. This fabulous superfood can be used to assist women with regulating their monthly cycle and decreasing the negative symptoms that are associated with a woman's menstrual cycle.

Many women suffer each month with heavy, uncomfortable menstrual periods, along with intense cramping, hormonal headaches, moodiness and the general feeling of not being well. If this is you or someone you know, I would highly recommend you begin adding Maca to your health regime to balance your system. Maca stimulates your own natural hormone production by promoting proper functioning of the pituitary gland and the hypothalamus. How simple is that? A fabulous superfood that creates balance in your body!

Because I have the joy of consulting with clients in my practice, as well as interacting with customers in my health food store, I have had many opportunities to discuss hormonal health with an abundance of women. These women are of all different sizes and ethnic backgrounds. What I learned from many of these women is that they believe an uncomfortable menstruation is just a part of life for them. They suffer through the symptoms each month using a pain-relieving drug such as Midol or Advil and go on with their life until their next cycle, experiencing an awful menstruation all over again.

I was shocked to find out that this was the normal reaction from the women I was speaking with about menstruation. This is completely unacceptable to me. Women were willing to simply suffer each month, feeling unwell and uncomfortable. These women had accepted the unpleasant experience of their monthly menstruation as normal.

I take the approach not only in my work but in my life that if you are not enjoying the experiences you are having, then you need to look at how you can improve them. To put it simply, you cannot expect a different outcome if you do not change your behavior.

Why not apply this way of thinking to your menstrual cycle? Yes, it is a fact that women are blessed with the ability to menstruate every month and I truly mean blessed. If your experience with menstruation each month is negative, then it is time to make a change. In addition to this point, if you suffer with uncomfortable and painful menstruation month after month, then it is time that you begin listening to your body as it is screaming at you for help!

I can assure you that the negative symptoms you are experiencing with menstruation are not due to the body being deficient in painkillers such as Midol or Advil. In fact, it is the exact opposite – your body is deficient in nutrients that are necessary to produce optimal functioning of your hormones, which would reduce the pain with menstruation.

Many of the women I introduce to Maca have not heard of this wonderful supplement and often feel it is too good to be true! The thought of pain free menstruation is completely unimaginable for them. It is hard for them to believe that with the regular use of Maca, you can greatly improve your monthly experience with menstruation.

TESTIMONIAL FROM SUE, AGE 46

*In the last few years, (perhaps the beginnings of peri-menapause?), I had started to experience strong PMS symptoms like anxiety, irritability, low energy and strong menstrual cramping and flow. Since starting to take Brad King's **Ultimate Maca Energy capsules** my symptoms have improved greatly. Not only has my anxiety and irritability diminished, but also I am sleeping better and have much more energy. There has also been an improvement in my menstrual flow and cramping. I recommend Brad King's **Ultimate Maca Energy capsules** to all my friends for any symptoms they may have, but also for more energy and an overall well-being.*

Including Maca in your daily health regime will provide the hormone balancing nutrients that your endocrine system is begging for and as a result will help create a balanced system. Being a practitioner of alternative health, I am still amazed that Maca has such incredible healing properties and that individuals can rebalance their bodies with the therapeutic use of this superfood.

Maca is a hormone regulator and therefore has the ability to stimulate the function of the endocrine hormones. As a hormone regulator, Maca can increase levels of estrogen, progesterone or testosterone naturally by nurturing the pituitary gland. The pituitary gland then instructs the necessary production of the hormones estrogen, progesterone or testosterone depending on the individuals needs. When you consume Maca regularly, the rich nutrients that naturally occur in this Peruvian superfood go to work on your endocrine system and create balance. Your only job is to remember to take your daily dose of Maca.

With time, you can have a balanced endocrine system with optimal hormone production. You can experience better moods, improved hormonal function and have balance during the time of menstruation.

TESTIMONIAL FROM NANCY, AGE 50

I started on my Maca adventure when my moods were getting a little hard to handle. Once a month for just a few days, the words that came flying out of my mouth shocked even me. I would stand there and think to myself 'Who just said that?' as I stood there stunned that I would have said something as nasty as I just did. I would walk away with the thoughts of 'What is wrong with me?' as I tried to recover from my shock. At that time, my cycle was not normal so these moods would hit at any time with no warning.

*When I heard about Maca I was willing to try anything to balance what was going on in my body. I started off with Brad King's **Ultimate Maca Energy capsules** and noticed the difference within a few weeks. My cycle was normal and there were no more mood swings, which I am sure everyone around me was quite happy about. Brad King's **Ultimate Maca Energy capsules** worked so quickly that I studied it to find out all I could about it. This amazing root from Peru is considered a 'Superfood' in the Rawfood movement (and I am a rawfoodist and provide lectures on the topic of raw food) so Maca quickly became part of my lectures. I loved the energy that I received from it and of course, the balancing of my hormones was the entire reason I started taking it.*

*I have since tried the **MacaPunch XP Platinum** liquid, which is excellent at giving immediate results and an amazing amount of energy. Right now, I have been using the **Ultimate Maca Energy powder** so that I can just add it to the smoothie I have every morning. I can increase the amount of powder I use if I feel that I need an extra amount. This 'Superfood' has energized and balanced my life!*

Try it for yourself!!

To improve your endocrine system and improve your menstrual cycle, it is important to consume the nutrients that the body is currently lacking. These nutrients will increase the production of the required hormones to create balance within the endocrine system. A balanced endocrine system makes for a happy menstruation…for everyone!

Maca Protocol:

Two teaspoons of **MacaPunch XP Platinum** liquid, three times a day, I would recommend that you remain at this dose for ninety days. If you prefer to use Brad King's **Ultimate Maca Energy capsules**, I would recommend six capsules, three times a day for ninety days. The female reproductive system takes time to rebalance and requires continuous nutrients for the system to correct itself.

After the ninety days, I recommend reducing your dosage to one teaspoon **MacaPunch XP Platinum** liquid twice daily or three capsules of Brad King's **Ultimate Maca Energy**, twice daily.

Then after an additional ninety days, I would reduce to one teaspoon a day of the **MacaPunch XP Platinum** liquid or three capsules of Brad King's **Ultimate Maca Energy** per day for maintenance.

You may find that throughout your cycle or at different times in your life (possibly in more stressful times) you may need to increase your dose of Maca. Listen to your body and adjust the dose as needed. The more balanced your endocrine system is, the better you will feel.

It is noteworthy that there are not any known side effects of taking Maca continuously. Maca is a superfood, not an artificial hormone, so it is very safe and effective for regular use.

Nutrition Tip:

In addition to taking Maca, diet is a very important factor to regulating hormones. To provide hormonal balance, it is necessary to consume quality foods such as whole grains, quality proteins, large servings of fruits and vegetables and small servings of healthy omega 3 fats. This whole foods approach to eating will provide your body with the necessary nutrients to build stamina and energy, as well as provide quality nutrients to promote a healthy hormonal system. For a complete guide of these suggested food groups, refer to *Appendix A; Introduction to a Whole Foods Lifestyle.*

Knowing which foods will promote health in your body is just as important as being aware of the foods that will hinder or not support your health.

There are certain categories of foods that are not beneficial to your hormonal health and should either be completely eliminated from your diet or severely reduced. Packaged and processed foods are very common "foods" that are severely over used. Packaged and processed foods should not be the staple of your diet, as they do not contain quality wholesome nutrients. Sweetners such as aspartame and white sugar are not quality foods and offer almost no vitamin or mineral content. As well, artificial preservatives and white flour products are "foods" that do not support the endocrine system or the production of healthy hormones. I placed quotations around food when referring to the list above because those categories are not real foods. The majority of the list is chemically made ingredients and therefore do not provide quality vitamins, minerals and nutrients that the endocrine system requires to function optimally. Always remember our bodies are made up of vitamins and minerals and that is the nutrient content that we require to function optimally. When we suffer with a symptom or an imbalance in our systems, we are not deficient in white flour, aspartame or preservatives – we are lacking nutrients. The symptoms we experience is our body's way of giving us a signal that we are nutrient deprived. It is then our responsibility to listen and take the appropriate action with quality nutrition and sensible supplementation to correct this imbalance.

Grocery Shopping Tip:
When reading food labels, it is important to focus on the first five ingredients of the nutrition label. If the first five ingredients contain, sugar, salt, a chemical or a word that you cannot pronounce, then this food is not of the quality that you want to support your hormonal system. The first five ingredients are the bulk of each product and if they are not actual foods,

then this product will not provide the nutritional support necessary for optimal function of your hormonal system. It is important that you are able to recognize each ingredient listed on the nutrition labels as a food.

TESTIMONIAL FROM DR. PIP, AGE 32

For as long as I can remember, I have had a short menstrual cycle, 21-24 days and my period lasting six full days. Even though I'm generally a very happy person, I still noticed, as did those around me, I was more easily frustrated and stressed in the week leading up to my period.
*I started taking **MacaPunch XP Platinum** liquid on Lorrie's recommendation and immediately saw my menstrual cycle lengthen that very month as well as only menstruating for five days or less.*
I also noticed that my mood swings were almost non-existent.

What a change in quality of life!
*I have since had several patients that I have referred to **MacaPunch XP Platinum** liquid for reproductive hormone help and for adrenal stress, and I have received only positive feedback. I can definitely say that **MacaPunch XP Platinum** liquid is now part of my healthy lifestyle!*

The Birth Control Pill and Maca

Another aspect of hormonal regulation is the use of the birth control pill in an attempt to balance a woman's hormones. Many women have used birth control pills to regulate their menstrual cycles and decrease the negative symptoms that are associated with a female's monthly menstruation. Before we go any further, I would like to discuss how the birth control pill works within a female body. The birth control pill provides the female body with artificial doses of the sex hormones estrogen and progesterone. These artificial hormones are designed to mimic the hormones that a women's body is naturally designed to produce. If a woman is experiencing an imbalanced endocrine system/hormonal system with symptoms such as painful menstruation, irregular cycles and moodiness, this indicates that her body is not producing the proper amount of estrogen and/or progesterone hormones. When this occurs, often the birth control pill is recommended to these women. The conventional medical profession uses birth control pills as a form of treatment to provide the female body with the required hormones to balance her endocrine system. Yes, this method can work to provide the necessary hormones that the female herself is not producing. However, this form of treatment does not uncover the root of the problem. Taking a synthetic form of hormones such as a birth control pill does not help the female's body to naturally begin production of her sex hormones estrogen and progesterone. Also, by taking a birth control pill to create hormone production, you still do not have the answer to why this woman is not able to properly produce her own hormones.

Maca is the answer to both of these concerns. The regular use of Maca will encourage the female body to increase production of the sex hormones estrogen and progesterone naturally. This method uncovers the root of the problem, (lack of hormone production) and provides a safe and natural solution. Dr. Hugo Malaspina, MD, prescribes Maca in his practice and his belief is "rather than introducing hormones from outside the body, Maca encourages the ovaries and other glands to produce the needed hormones." (Hilgan Enterprise Inc.).

Using a birth control pill and providing synthetic forms of estrogen and progesterone to the body creates a variety of changes in a women's reproductive system. The goal of the birth control pill is to stop ovulation or inhibit the release of an egg from the women's ovaries to essentially prevent pregnancy. When taking a birth control pill, the medication provides you with a prescribed amount of the synthetic hormones estrogen and progesterone. A side effect of taking the birth control pill is the possibility of the uterus lining becoming thin over time. If and when a female decides that she wants to conceive a child, the uterus lining could potentially be too thin due to the use of the birth control pill, making it difficult for a fertilized egg to implant into the uterus lining (www.epigee.org). Another side effect from taking the birth control pill is what is referred to as post pill amenorrhea. Post pill amenorrhea is when the "birth control pill prevents your body from making hormones involved in ovulation and menstruation" even after you are no longer taking the birth control pill. (http://www.mayoclinic.com/health/birth-control-pill/WO00098).

When a female stops the use of the birth control pill, it can take some time for her endocrine system to return to normal and begin producing hormones naturally. At this time, the female is considered infertile as her body has not begun the natural production of her sex hormones. As a result, the woman will not ovulate and at this time cannot conceive a child. A sign that the female is naturally producing hormones is ovulation and menstruation. For some women, this process of regulating the endocrine system can take anywhere from three to six months after she has stopped the use of the birth control pill. The above side effects are created from providing the body with synthetic forms of estrogen and progesterone – all to regulate a woman's menstrual cycle. I have a better solution to regulate a woman's menstrual cycle. It is safe, natural, effective and can be used confidently knowing there are not any known side effects. This wonderful solution is MACA!

Now, before we discuss the wonderful benefits that Maca can provide to the female reproductive system, I think it is important to examine the way in which we look at the imbalances in women's health. I think it is important to discover why so many women's bodies are not producing the required sex hormones? It is very common for woman to have a menstrual cycle out of balance and the first response should be, Why is my body not balanced? Why am I not producing the necessary hormones to provide balance to my reproductive system?

Irregular menstruation, heavy flow and intense cramping are some of the symptoms associated with menstruation for some women each and every month. These symptoms are not occurring because the body is lacking the artificial hormones found in a birth control pill. The reason a female may experience these symptoms is because her hormonal system is not balanced. She is not naturally producing the required estrogen and progesterone to regulate her menstrual cycle and eliminate these unpleasant symptoms. As a holistic practitioner, I believe it is important to find the source of the problem and truly correct the imbalance so the body can function optimally. My question is why are so many women not creating the hormones required to have a healthy menstrual cycle and can this imbalance be corrected? And my answer is Absolutely!

As I discussed earlier in the book, a woman's role today is much more demanding and has created a higher level of daily stress. With more stress and possibly suffering with Adrenal Fatigue comes a compromised endocrine system. Women are not providing enough care to themselves, by replenishing their hormonal systems. (Refer to Lifestyle Suggestions in section on Adrenal Fatigue & Maca). A combination of high stress, poor diet and not enough relaxation time has created an imbalance within the female endocrine system. As we have examined, when there is an imbalance within the endocrine system, adequate levels of hormones are not produced. As a result, the female body then suffers with ongoing hormone imbalances such as uncomfortable and unpleasant menstruation. The good news is YES, this imbalance can be corrected with the wonderful superfood MACA!

Dr. Chacon, Maca expert, stated in *Nature & Health Magazine* (December 1999 January 2000) "It is important to remember that Maca does not contain any hormones but its action in the body jogs the pituitary (gland) into producing the precursor hormones, which ultimately end up raising estrogen, progesterone and testosterone levels, as well as helping to balance the adrenal glands, the thyroid and the pancreas."

The superfood Maca can improve hormonal imbalance and provide women with a solution to their ongoing battle with their endocrine system. Maca is a natural way to balance a female's hormones without side effects. This superfood is safe, natural and effective. Maca provides the body the ability to create the hormones naturally that the female's endocrine system is struggling to produce. As well, using Maca instead of a synthetic birth control pill (to regulate a female hormonal cycle) will provide women with the quality nutrients their endocrine system is lacking. Once the system is balanced, the body is able to set up the reproductive system to conceive a child when and if the woman so chooses.

Maca and the birth control pill are not one hundred percent interchangeable. If you are taking the birth control pill to prevent the conception of a child, then please note that Maca does not prevent pregnancy. Maca assists with increasing the female's hormones to balance the endocrine system and helps to improve uncomfortable menstruation and promote menstrual regulation. The birth control pill is used to correct hormonal imbalances and is designed to prevent conception of a fetus. Maca does not prevent conception of a fetus. In fact, Maca increases the chances of fertility. So keep in mind if you are looking for a natural approach to balancing your hormones, Maca can greatly assist with that process. However, if you are also looking for a product to prevent pregnancy, remember that Maca will not prevent pregnancy, as that is not what it is designed to do.

TESTIMONIAL FROM LYNN, AGE 42

I was on a birth control pill to control my periods and went off because I was gaining weight. When I got my period again, I was very sick, very grouchy and in a lot of pain. Lorrie suggested I take Brad King's **Ultimate Maca Energy capsules** *to help, after taking it for about for a month I improved a lot. My moods have improved, and the pain has decreased. Thank you so much Lorrie for suggesting Maca. It is a life saver.*

Maca Protocol:

One teaspoon of **MacaPunch XP Platinum** liquid, three times daily or three capsules of Brad King's **Ultimate Maca Energy capsules**, three times daily.

Nutrition Tip:

Consuming foods from a whole foods lifestyle will increase your overall well-being. Eliminating white flour products along with packaged and processed food will keep your system more balanced and therefore provide more nutrient support to your hormonal system. (Refer to *Appendix A- Introduction to a Whole Foods Lifestyle* for a complete guideline).

Female Fertility and Maca

Fertility is defined as the "ability to conceive and have children, the ability to become pregnant through normal sexual activity" (www.medterms.com). Conversely, infertility is defined as "the diminished ability or the inability to conceive and have offspring. Infertility is also defined in specific terms as "the failure to conceive after a year of regular intercourse without contraception." (www.medterms.com) The topic of fertility is very popular and is always surrounded with many questions and concerns.

According to Beverly Hanck, the executive director of the Infertility Awareness Association of Canada, couples should begin planning families in their twenties. (www.thehealthjournal.ca) "Young women fail to realize that their fertility starts declining from their mid-to late twenties. Currently, one in every six to eight couples of reproductive age will have difficulty conceiving." *The Health Journal* states "By the time a women is thirty-five, her conception rate will decline by fifty per cent; miscarriage and genetic abnormality rates also increase with age."

A female's role can be very demanding in our current society. Many women work not only within their home but also have a full time career outside of the home. The lifestyle that many women live today is very high pace, with many deadlines, and try to be everything to everyone. This type of lifestyle can be a contributing factor within the issue of infertility. When an individual is stressed or very busy without any relaxation time, this can have a very negative impact on the body. Often, when prolonged periods of stress are held within the body, this can create hormonal imbalances. As discussed in sections Stress and Maca, as well as Adrenal Fatigue and Maca, when the body reaches a point of physical, mental and emotional exhaustion, the stress glands (known as the adrenal glands) become overwhelmed and decrease their ability to function. When the adrenals glands are not functioning optimally, this creates an imbalance within the endocrine system/ hormonal system. When a woman is trying to conceive a child and there is an imbalance in her hormonal system, this makes the goal of conceiving a child very challenging and can contribute to the issue of infertility. This same scenario in terms of an unbalanced hormonal system can occur in men. If men are overworked, stressed and suffering with Adrenal Fatigue, they too will have a decrease in the production of their sex hormone testosterone. This can contribute to low sperm production and make creating a baby more challenging. (Refer to section on Men and Maca for further details on infertility in men and the use of Maca).

"From 1979 to 1999, the fertility of Canadian women aged twenty to twenty-four decreased nearly forty per cent and fertility among those aged twenty-five to twenty-nine declined by twenty-five per cent." (StatsCanada, www.statcan.gc.ca). According to Statistics Canada, the average age a woman gives birth to her first child is nearly twenty-nine years of age. This confirms that even though statistically the female reproductive system is optimal in a woman's early twenties, Canadian women are still choosing to begin their families almost ten to fifteen years later than the suggested optimal age of fertility. Many women are attending college or university after high school, establishing their career, focusing on marriage and then beginning a family.

As women begin creating their families much later, many report the ideal time in their life to conceive a child does not coincide with the age range that fertility experts recommend. Many women find that it does take longer than they expected to conceive a child as fertility experts report. The struggle to become pregnant can be attributed to a couple of factors,the first one being the age, as already mentioned. As a woman ages, her chances of conceiving a child significantly decreases. Secondly, if a woman struggles with imbalanced hormones, it seems logical that before she can conceive a child, she will need to balance her endocrine system. Without balancing her hormones, conceiving a child may be very difficult and, as a result, a very disappointing process.

Many women find themselves in this situation. The female and her partner have decided they want to begin their family and the woman discovers that she has an imbalance within her endocrine system. This can delay the process of beginning a family until the woman is able to balance her hormones within her endocrine system. The imbalance may not necessarily be due to the low production of estrogen or progesterone, but in fact could be an imbalanced adrenal gland, or an under-active thyroid. If these glands are not functioning optimally and producing the required amounts of hormones, then the endocrine system will be out of balance. This too can create issues when trying to conceive a child.

With all the possible contributing factors listed above, I do not mean to imply that a woman between the ages of thirty and forty will have great difficulty conceiving a child. The information provided is to assist you to be aware that there are many imbalances that can occur within the body that have an effect on fertility. It is important to realize that when all of the glands within the endocrine system work in unison and produce their required hormones, a very healthy and inviting environment can be created for conceiving a child.

The introduction of Maca to an unbalanced endocrine system can greatly assist with increasing the female's hormone production, energize exhausted adrenals and provide support to an underactive thyroid, even when a woman is past the optimal age for fertility.

When dealing with the possibility of infertility, it is important to provide quality nutrients to the endocrine system as stress will be elevated with any couple struggling to conceive a child without success.

Consuming Maca regularly is imperative to provide the adaptogenic and hormone-balancing healing benefits. Maca provides not only the correct nutrients to support the production of hormones to improve fertility, but Maca is also a nutrient-rich food that will support the nervous system due to the stress related to this situation.

When dealing with fertility issues, it is ideal for both partners to be consuming high levels of the superfood Maca. The male can also take the same dose recommended in the protocol below.

Research supports that Maca has positive effects on men and their endocrine system. Maca can increase the hormone testosterone, the motility of sperm and assist with increasing sperm production. As well, it is important that we support the male's adrenal gland, better known as the stress gland. Both partners will be suffering from underlying stress of trying to conceive. (Refer to *Men and Maca* for a more detailed description of the healing benefits of Maca with men).

Maca can assist to regulate all the possibilities of infertility that I have mentioned in this book. WOW! What an incredible product… and that it is!

A **SPECIAL NOTE**; if you have been taking Maca before you conceived a child and feel that you will need hormonal support throughout your pregnancy, there are no known side effects of taking Maca while pregnant. Remember; this is a superfood that regulates your hormones. Woman in Peru continue their use of Maca during pregnancy and even while breast feeding their newborns. If you are unsure or wish to discuss using Maca during pregnancy, I would recommend you contact a holistic health practitioner who is familiar with the healing benefits of Maca. Although there is not any research supporting Maca as harmful during pregnancy, I would not recommend you begin a supplement regime with Maca if you are pregnant and were not using Maca prior to becoming pregnant. I would recommend the same advice for any nutritional supplement. Once you know you are pregnant, I would not introduce any new supplements until after the baby is born and you are no longer breastfeeding.

Maca Protocol:
One teaspoon of **MacaPunch XP Platinum** liquid, six times daily, or three capsules of Brad King's **Ultimate Maca Energy**, six times day.

Nutrition Tip:

If you are at the stage in your life that you are trying to begin a family and if you have not already embraced the idea of a whole foods lifestyle, I would recommend that you begin right now. If you are trying to create a new life, then it is ideal to provide this new being with optimal nutrients. Refer to *Appendix A; Introduction to a Whole Food Lifestyle* for a complete description of what food groups are included in this way of eating.

When creating optimal health, it is important that you are not consuming high processed and packaged foods. As previously stated, these foods offer very few nutrients and can also create inflammation within the body due to the high saturated fats, high salt and high sugar content.

When trying to build a healthy environment for a baby to grow, it is important that you decrease the stimulants that you ingest such as caffeine, artificial sweetners, aspartame and regular soda as well as diet soda. Choose more natural sweetners such as sucanat (evaporated cane juice). These will provide your body with better blood sugar regulation, which will then provide a better foundation for hormonal balance.

When you are preparing to conceive a child, keep in mind that the foods you eat are going to be the nutrients that feed the baby while the baby is developing. If the foods you are choosing to eat are not wholesome, and healthy or not rich in nutrients, then remove them from your diet and focus on better quality foods. A woman is essentially the host for a growing fetus, so as the host, you want to create the most nutrient-rich environment possible.

Other Nutrient Recommendations:

When you are trying to conceive a child, be sure that you are taking a quality prenatal multi-vitamin. Taking a multi-vitamin will allow your body to build up stores of quality nutrients that you may be lacking in your diet. I recommend my clients take a prenatal multi-vitamin for at least three months prior to conceiving a child to provide the necessary nutrients to the woman's body to prepare as a host for a developing fetus.

I would also recommend that you begin taking a quality omega 3 nutritional supplement. Supplementing with omega 3 is very important for cognition and brain development in a developing fetus. It is ideal for the mother to have an abundance of omega 3 oils for the baby to draw from while developing. It is just as important for Mom to receive this nutrient to keep her hormonal system balanced during pregnancy.

It is ideal to begin taking an omega 3 supplement approximately three months prior to becoming pregnant to allow the woman to have optimal omega 3 stores at the time of conception.

I would highly recommend **Renew Life's Ultimate Fish Oils – Super Critical Omega**.

Visit your local health food store for these essential supplements.

With poor food choices such as a diet high in sugars and processed foods, there can be an issue with a condition of an over-production of yeast called candida albicans. Candida albicans "is a type of fungus, a mircroorganism that is not beneficial for the body; therefore, it is called "unfriendly" bacteria."(*Complete Candida Yeast Guidebook*, revised Second Addition, Martin, Jeanne, Marie, 2000, pg 1). A reproductive system with an over-production of yeast can create high levels of inflammation and produce an unhealthy environment for a fetus to survive. Candida yeast can bind to hormones in the body and hinder them from completing their job. It can also create false hormones, tricking the body into thinking proper hormone production is occurring, when in fact it is not. This creates an imbalance within the endocrine system and can wreak havoc with the entire functioning of the individual's body. I have seen numerous times in my practice where women who struggle with candida, struggle with fertility issues as well. With this being a common situation I see in my practice, I recommend, the following solution, along with following the Maca protocol outlined above.

To remove Candida from the system, it is important to conduct a quality candida cleanse. **Renew Life-Candigone Cleanse** would be ideal as this cleanse will rid the body of the yeast overgrowth.

If a woman has suffered with yeast issues since she began menstruating or if she suffers with more than three vaginal yeast infections per year, I recommend conducting the **Renew Life Candigone cleansing kit** for one to three months. This length of time will assist in removing the over-production of yeast and any congestion that may be occurring within her reproductive system due to this imbalance. With **Renew Life Candigone cleansing kit**, there is a suggested meal plan, be sure to follow the guidelines and you will see great results.

If you are pregnant or become pregnant while taking this cleanse, stop the cleanse immediately. Cleansing releases toxins and is not beneficial to a growing fetus.

Menopause and Maca

From the time of birth until her last day on earth, a women's body is constantly going through various hormonal changes. The final big hormonal change that women experience is what is referred to as the "change of life" or menopause. This change can actually occur at any age. Reports have been as early as thirty years old, however the average age in western society is fifty-one years of age. As with every hormonal change, it is unique to each woman, so it is important to note that there is not a set age, but simply a guideline as to what has occurred in the majority of women. How well balanced a woman has been hormonally throughout her life may have an impact on her experience with menopause. If a woman's experience has been a balanced hormonal system with regular menstruation and minimal discomfort, then menopause may not be a negative experience. However, if a woman has always suffered with hormonal imbalances and unpleasant menstrual symptoms, then menopause may be equally as uncomfortable.

During my research, I found it very interesting that women all over the world report very different experiences with menopause, in particular the women of Peru. These women do not suffer the severe menopausal symptoms nor do they dread the awful change of life with night sweats, weight gain and day time hot flashes. The women of Peru are hormonally balanced and do not experience menopause the way western women do. It is very interesting that women in the western world suffer so intensely with unbalanced hormonal systems while women in another country do not experience anything comparable.

This leads me to the question; what is the secret the women of Peru know, that women of western societies do not? The answer is MACA! Let's take a look at the topic of menopause and how Maca can help.

The conventional medical system reports a woman is going through menopause when she begins to experience irregular menstrual cycles, along with hot flashes, vaginal dryness, moodiness and a low sex drive. Conventional medicine believes that a woman has completed menopause when she has not experienced her menstrual cycle for twelve consecutive months, thus marking the completion of the woman's fertility and child-bearing abilities. In terms of hormone production, "natural menopause occurs when the ovaries naturally begin decreasing their production of the sex hormones estrogen and progesterone" (www.medterms.com).

As previously mentioned, menopause is often perceived as an unpleasant change in life for women in the western world. This negative outlook is not because it symbolizes the end of fertility but because of the multiple unpleasant physical symptoms that many women experience during "the change." It is normal for the female body to go through hormonal changes. In fact it is part of development and maturation. However, it is not intended to be perceived as a disease or a negative health condition.

Menopause is a hormonal transition that can be corrected by providing balance to the endocrine system.

When focused on balancing the endocrine system, I believe that women can reach this time in their lives and celebrate this transition, feel well and not suffer with these negative symptoms. I believe the symptoms that result from hormonal imbalance can be corrected. To correct a hormonal imbalance the individual must commit to discovering the root cause and then take action to correct their system with healthy lifestyle choices such as nutrition and sensible supplementation.

There are different options for women going through menopause; hormone replacement therapy, the use of natural supplements such as Black Cohosh or incorporating the superfood Maca! I bet you can already guess my favourite solution!

Hormone replacement therapy (HRT) is prescribed by a medical doctor and is the use of synthetic hormones. The female is prescribed these synthetic hormones to alleviate the negative symptoms associated with menopause. With continual use of these synthetic hormones, the endocrine system will eventually stop trying to produce the body's natural hormones estrogen and progesterone. The body will rely on the synthetic hormones for every day hormone production. This was the treatment of choice many years ago. However, research has revealed that there are more risks than benefits to this form of treatment. The National Institute of Health conducted studies to evaluate the risk and benefits to HRT. The results revealed the following: in one year of using HRT, there was an increase in coronary heart disease, stroke, blood clots in the lungs and legs and more cases of invasive breast cancer within the women using the HRT compared to the placebo group (www.hc-sc. gc.ca/hl-vs/iyh-vsv/med/estrogen-eng.php). The results of these studies alarmed many women and forced them to begin seeking out a more natural and alternative treatment for balancing their hormones during menopause.

In regards to natural and alternative approaches to decrease the symptoms of menopause, there are two options. The first one is the use of herbal remedies such as black cohosh. Black cohosh is an herb that is thought to possibly have phytoestrogenic properties. This means the use of black cohosh could mimic that of the hormone estrogen. A natural supplement that contains phytoestrogenic herbs essentially provides the body with a natural form of estrogen and there have been reports of its success with reducing hot flashes. With the prolonged use of phytoestrogenic herbs, it has been noted that the body can become less responsive to producing estrogen on its own. This is a result of the body getting used to being supplied with estrogen from a nutritional supplement such as black cohosh. This approach is very similar to HRT in that the body relies on an outside source to provide the estrogen for hormonal balance. In this instance, the source is a nutritional supplement, not a chemical like HRT. As well, black cohosh does not have the many negative side effects that were identified with conventional HRT. There are still mixed results when it comes to black cohosh and its beneficial effects on menopause.

Another natural approach to menopause and balancing hormones is the use of Maca, a non-estrogenic herb. Non-estrogenic herbs do not contain estrogen, but instead provide nourishment to the endocrine glands, so they are able to work efficiently and produce their own hormones in the necessary amounts. This form of nutritional supplement is the most natural way to encourage the production of hormones within the human body. Maca is well known as an overall hormone balancer and it is very effective in reducing the symptoms associated with menopause such as hot flashes, moodiness and the decrease in sex drive. The use of Maca is a very safe and effective way to reduce the symptoms of menopause, as well as restoring balance to the entire endocrine system.

Hormonally speaking, menopause is the decrease of the sex hormones estrogen and progesterone. It is important to provide the body with nutrients that will assist with balancing these decreasing hormones and not allow them to reduce too quickly.

The amazing superfood and nutritional supplement Maca can provide just what the body is looking for in terms of hormone regulation. Maca aids in the natural production of the body's estrogen and progesterone. Maca is a hormonal regulator. When taken consistently, Maca will provide the body with the required nutrients to increase the levels of estrogen and progesterone that are decreasing during menopause. With Maca being a non-estrogenic superfood, this food supplement is a safe and natural way to balance the endocrine system and reduce the negative symptoms associated with menopause.

There is nothing artificial about Maca or the process that it promotes within a woman's hormonal system. Nourishing the hormonal system with the regular use of Maca is simply orchestrating communication within the endocrine system and making menopause more of a pleasant transition than a horrible hormonal experience.

Research has shown that Maca does not contain plant hormones but in fact relies on the naturally occurring plant sterols. Plant sterols act as chemical triggers to assist the body to produce higher levels of hormones that are necessary to not only the individual's age but also their gender.

With the increase in production of these hormones, women going through the change of life or menopause can be confident that Maca will assist to reduce their symptoms of hot flashes, moodiness and a low sex drive.

TESTIMONIAL FROM ANNE, AGE 54

*I have been taking Maca for a little over a year and have found that I don't have very many hot flashes, not like before when I would have several in a day. I am taking the **MacaPunch XP Platinum** liquid which is an acquired taste and not for the weak as it has a taste all its own. Also, when you have the afternoon slump, a spoonful of the **MacaPunch XP Platinum** liquid and you have energy to burn, life is good.*

Another symptom many menopausal woman report is trouble sleeping at night. This is also due to the imbalance within the body's hormones. Many women report waking at night in wet clothes from their hot flashes, then they are not able to fall back to sleep once they have cooled down. As a result, by morning they are not feeling well rested and are in fact moody due to their sleepless night. If the sleepless nights are related to the woman's imbalanced hormonal system, then her sleep will improve with the regular use of Maca. As well, she will experience a reduction in hot flashes and her moodiness will turn to a more pleasant state of mind.

Women have reported a reduction in their hot flashes within two to three days after they begin taking Maca. However, other women have stated that it took up to six weeks to see noticeable results. Hormone balancing is very individual and it is important to understand that your hormones did not suddenly become out of balance within a day, or even a week, so it could take some time to get them organized again. Also keep in mind each person is an individual, so be patient and consistent and you will be pleased with the results. And before you know it, you will be recommending Maca to all your friends!

Maca Protocol:

One teaspoon of **MacaPunch XP Platinum** Liquid, four times daily or three capsules of Brad King's **Ultimate Maca Energy** four times daily for twelve weeks.

Within twelve weeks you should notice a significant reduction in your menopausal symptoms. At that point, reduce your intake of **MacaPunch XP Platinum** liquid to one teaspoon, three times daily, or three capsules of Brad King's **Ultimate Maca Energy** three times daily for four weeks.

After the four weeks, reduce your dosage to one teaspoon of **MacaPunch XP Platinum** liquid, twice daily or three capsules of Brad King's **Ultimate Maca Energy**, twice daily. You can remain at this dose as your maintenance dose.

If you find that you begin reducing the dosage and your menopausal symptoms return, then increase the dose for an additional four weeks. Try to reduce the dose after four weeks again. Everyone's bodies and hormones may require a slightly different dose, so be comfortable with adjusting your intake of Maca to provide balance to your system and eliminate your symptoms.

Nutrition Tip:

Along with supplementing the hormonal system with the superfood Maca, the quality of food you consume does play a role in women's hot flashes and menopausal symptoms. In my nutritional consulting practice, many women have reported that once they eliminated white flour and processed sugar from their diet, they noticed a significant improvement in the intensity of their hot flashes. (Refer to *Appendix A for the*

Introduction to a Whole Foods Lifestyle to provide you with a guideline to healthy hormonal eating).

Even though hot flashes and menopausal symptoms are an imbalance within the hormonal system, foods such as white flour, white sugar, packaged and processed foods all can have a negative impact on the hormonal system and add to the intensity of the hot flashes. These foods do not provide rich nutrients to support the hormonal system. In fact, these foods are void of nutrients and create an imbalance, often resulting in the individual struggling with blood sugar imbalances. When this occurs, the individual begins to crave the unhealthy foods more often, as the body is in need of sugar. A solution to that ongoing battle is to incorporate three to five servings of quality protein in your daily diet. (Refer to Appendix B for a list of quality protein sources).

Be sure to include a serving of protein at breakfast, mid-morning snack (approximately 10:00-10:30am), lunch, mid-afternoon snack (2:30-3:00pm) and at your supper meal. If you can improve your diet along with taking the superfood Maca, you will greatly reduce your symptom of hot flashes, along with increasing your energy and vitality.

TESTIMONIAL FROM DOROTHY, AGE 47

*Maca... a couple of years ago I started the next stage in life – the dreaded menopause. The hot flashes – going from blood boiling, wanting to tear off my clothes, taking a shower because the sweat is rolling down every where, to putting on a sweater because you're now cold. Then there is the mood swings – the lows to the very low feeling where I wanted to cry a river to feeling like every person is standing on your last nerve and wishing that I could just hide from the world. After taking **MacaPunch XP Platinum** liquid, menopause is not so bad. My moods are better – I have warm flashes once in a while but they are much more tolerable. **MacaPunch XP Platinum** liquid has also helped with my menstrual migraines. I rarely get them anymore. I'm sure if you ask my three nieces (aged 19, 20 and 22), they would probably thank Maca as well – after being "trapped" in a automobile with me for 24 hours for our road trip to and from Dallas to visit my oldest sister. We really had a fantastic time! So thanks Lorrie for taming the Hulk in me! It really helped.*

Andropause and Maca

It was once believed that only women went through menopause or "change of life" and experienced a shift in their hormones. However, research supports that in fact men also experience a shift in hormones later in life and it is called Andropause. Andropause is not directly comparable to women in menopause because andropause can be a more gradual process occurring over ten to fifteen years on average for most men. For women, menopause often occurs between mid-forties to mid-fifties and is triggered by the lack of menstruation. Another difference is women have an indication with the cessation of their menstrual cycle that their hormones are shifting within their system. However, men do not have one distinguishing factor that tells them their hormonal system is changing. Often, because there is not one specific factor, andropause can go undiagnosed. Men will often be treated for depression and anxiety disorders or simply feel the decrease in their energy is acceptable with age. The one similarity between the two genders is that menopause and andropause are both related to a decrease in hormonal activity for men and women.

This concept of andropause is not a new phenomenon. In fact andropause was first described in medical literature in the 1940's. Our ability to diagnose and recognize these symptoms as a hormonal imbalance is what has improved. Many men have gone undiagnosed with hormonal imbalances for many years. Now, with men living longer and demanding a better quality of life, this imbalance has been detected and is now being recognized and treated.

For men, andropause indicates that the male's hormonal system is not producing as much testosterone as it once did. Or it is producing significantly less testosterone than is required to maintain a balanced hormonal system.

The hormone testosterone is crucial to men's health. It stimulates sexual development in male infants, as well as assists to develop bone. Testosterone is also responsible for muscle growth, strength and stamina in males as they mature. Testosterone is the prominent hormone in males during the time of puberty and this hormone is responsible for growth of facial and genital hair, along with the deepening of the male's voice. Testosterone is also responsible for the male's sex drive. As you can see, testosterone plays a critical role in the function of the male's body from infant through puberty and into their senior years.

A males' testosterone levels increase at the time of puberty and remain fairly consistent until the age of thirty. Research supports that a male's testosterone levels begin to decrease around the age of thirty and at this age, a male's testosterone levels can drop as much as one to two per cent annually (http://www.sciencedaily.com/releases/2010/05/100514171916. htm). This means that every decade, a male's testosterones levels can reduce ten to twenty per cent. With a male's testosterone levels decreasing at this rapid rate, by the time a man reaches the age of forty to fifty-five years old, he could be experiencing what we now know as andropause.

The symptoms related to andropause can be any or all of the following; lethargy, depression, increased irritability, mood swings, hot flashes (the sweats), insomnia, decreased libido, weakness, loss of lean body mass, and difficulty attaining and sustaining erections (impotence), increased body fat, osteoporosis and even cardiovascular risk. According to the *American Journal of Hypertenstion*, (1999;12;271-275) forty to sixty per cent percent of men suffer with some symptoms of andropause.

Research supports that even healthy men can see a significant decrease in testosterone levels. By the age of fifty, the amount of testosterone secreted into the blood stream of a man is significantly lower than ten to fifteen years earlier. By the age of eighty years, many male's hormonal levels will have decreased to pre-puberty levels (www.ahealthya.com).

Besides hormonal deficiencies, there are other known contributing factors that play a role in andropause; excessive alcohol consumption, smoking, hypertension, prescription and non-prescription drugs, poor diet, lack of exercise and poor circulation.

Similar to women and menopause, men from outside of western society do not suffer with this condition of andropause. As I asked in the case of women and menopause, I have to ask – what are the men in other countries doing that is different? Or even more important – what are men in western society lacking? A good example is the men of Peru. These men do not have such a drastic decrease in testosterone levels in their male population. In fact, the men of Peru are sexually active without any medications well into their eighties. Their testosterone levels remain healthy and high which enables them to function better as they have more lean body mass, more stamina, a healthier libido and an abundance of energy when compared to men of other societies. The reason for this discrepancy in the two countries is the men of Peru consume Maca root on a regular basis and use it as a staple in their diet. Maca is high in amino acids and acts as a hormone regulator, providing the body with optimal levels of the necessary hormones for energy and sex drive. The Peruvian male's testosterone levels remain high as they are consuming the required nutrients to produce optimal levels of this important hormone, testosterone.

Maca Protocol:

One teaspoon of **MacaPunch XP Platinum** Liquid, four times daily, or three capsules of Brad King's **Ultimate Maca Energy** four times daily for twelve weeks.

Within twelve weeks, you should notice a significant reduction in your andropause symptoms. At that point, reduce your intake of **MacaPunch XP Platinum** liquid to one teaspoon, three times daily or three capsules of Brad King's **Ultimate Maca Energy** three times a day for four weeks.

After the four weeks, reduce your dosage to one teaspoon of **MacaPunch XP Platinum** liquid, twice daily or three capsules of Brad King's **Ultimate Maca Energy** twice daily.

You can remain at this dose as your maintenance dose.

Nutrition Tip:

In addition to the Maca protocol, diet is a crucial part of balancing the hormonal system. With poor diet being one the contributing factors to andropause, I would highly recommend a whole foods approach to nutrition. (Refer to *Appendix A for guidelines on the Introduction to a Whole Food Lifestyle*).

As well, I would recommend that you limit the intake of saturated fats such as red meat, pork and fried foods. I would recommend to focus more on the good fats listed in *Appendix A- Introduction to a Whole Foods Lifestyle.* Good fats support a healthy hormonal system and that is one of the crucial nutrients lacking when the male body suffers with symptoms of andropause.

Grocery Tip:

Each time you go to the grocery store, buy a product that is considered a whole foods product. For example, next grocery trip instead of buying white bread, try one of the many whole grain breads available. In no time, you will be able to replace all the nutrient-depleted foods that stock your kitchen, with nutrient rich foods that will stock your body full of energy!

Aphrodisiac Activity, Libido and Maca

In today's society, a decreased sex drive in both men and women is a common complaint. In a review of low libido and women, the *International Journal of STD & AIDS* reported, "Low libido is the most frequently reported sexual dysfunction." There are many factors that play a role in low libido in both men and women. One area is the imbalance within the hormonal system and the inadequate supply of sex hormones being produced resulting in a decrease in both men and women's sex drive.

In my health food store, I discuss this very topic with many couples. When these individuals come to my store for advice, they feel embarrassed and sometimes find it very difficult to discuss their symptoms. Once I am able to educate them on what is happening in their body and they realize they are suffering with a hormonal imbalance, they have a better understanding of their situation. They no longer think there is something wrong with them. Their self-confidence increases again when I explain to them the benefits of using Maca, a safe and natural libido enhancer.

Do you recall when I explained what it means when we have a symptom? It means that we are lacking specific nutrients within our system and as a result a symptom has been created to inform us of this imbalance.

This is the case with low libido; the male or female's body is not consuming the required nutrients to provide optimal hormone production. When the male's body is not producing enough testosterone and the female's body is not producing enough estrogen, this can result in low libido or loss of sex drive.

With the regular use of Maca the body is absorbing rich nutrients that support and feed the endocrine system which instructs production of the sex hormones testosterone and estrogen. With the increase in the hormone production, this promotes an increase in sex drive in both men and women.

Many Canadians use this power-packed food in supplement form and its most popular use is as a hormone balancer. Maca is not a synthetic drug or a medication. It is a food that contains rich nutrients which enhance the body's ability to increase the necessary hormones to provide balance to the overall system. This superfood is beneficial and necessary to any individual who struggles with an imbalanced hormonal system.

In a three month trial with twelve male volunteers, a scientist named Gonzales of Peru's Cayetano Heredia University reported a 180 to 200 per cent increase in libido and up to double the increase in sperm production. The men reported an increase in their sex drive, just two weeks after taking between 3000 and 5000mg of Maca for this study (Hilgan Enterprises Inc).

As previously mentioned, in the time of the Incas Warriors, the men were given Maca before they went to battle to assist with keeping their bodies strong and equipped for intense physical activity. While taking Maca, the men noticed an increase in their libido and upon return from battle, the warriors were forbidden to take Maca in order to protect the women from the men's sexual impulses. In the time of the Incas, the act of sex and the action of sexuality was portrayed very differently than today. Consuming Maca today will not make you a sexual deviant as was portrayed in the time of the Incas. Consuming Maca regularly will in fact increase a low sex drive to a healthy state of sexual desire.

Chemical research supports that Maca root naturally contains a chemical – p-methoxybenzyl isothisocyanate – which is responsible for the aphrodisiac properties and the increase in sex drive in both men and women.

The International Journal of Urology published a study in which they gave an oral administration of a purified lipidic extract from Lepidium Meyenii (Maca) to mating mice. The results produced were an enhanced sexual function in the mice. This study revealed an increase in aphrodisiac activity due to the consumption of Lepidium Meyenii (Maca).

Additional research supports that Maca not only increases sexual desire and is an aphrodisiac but when taken regularly, it is also known to improve male potency in terms of sperm production, as well as aid in erectile dysfunction. These imbalances in men are related to a low level of testosterone. Adequate levels of testosterone are necessary to maintain a healthy sex drive, to promote muscle growth, to develop and maintain an erection and also for the male's emotional and psychological development.

TESTIMONIAL FROM HUGH, AGE 53

I began taking **MacaPunch XP Platinum** *liquid about two years ago. When I first began using* **MacaPunch XP Platinum** *liquid, I was taking one teaspoon daily. After a short time, I noticed I had more energy both physically and mentally, I felt sharper and was experiencing more mental clarity. I noticed an overall increase in my general well-being. As I learned more about Maca, I realized I could increase my dose significantly, so I did. I now take between six and nine teaspoons daily and I have noticed an increase in my libido, as well as an increase in the benefits that I was already experiencing.*

Maca Protocol (for both men and women):

One teaspoon of **MacaPunch XP Platinum** liquid, four to six times daily or three capsules of Brad King's **Ultimate Maca Energy**, four to six times daily.

The dosage of Maca required for increase in libido will depend on how deficient the hormonal stores are within each individual. This is a protocol that you will need to work with and discover what is best suited to increase your personal sex drive.

Nutrition Tip:

When it comes to nutrition and increasing sex drive, the best advice is to eat a clean, wholesome healthy diet. If you are noticing that your body is not producing optimally, such as an imbalance within your hormones, it is best to begin eating well. The better the quality of food you take in, the more balanced and nutrient-rich your body becomes.

Begin incorporating a whole foods diet refer to *Appendix A- Introduction to a Whole Food Lifestyle.*

Include four to five servings of quality protein daily (one serving is equivalent to 3 oz). Consistent intake of protein will assist with balancing your blood sugar level. Refer to *Appendix B* for a list of Protein Sources.

This means you will not crave sugars and breads. Creating a body that has balanced blood sugar levels provide more nutritional support to the hormonal system.

Eliminate any processed stimulants such as coffee, energy drinks, sugar or other caffeine drinks. Regular use of these foods will create stress within the hormonal system and as a result create an imbalance.

19

Erectile Dysfunction and Maca

According to the Canadians Men's Clinic Limited, an estimated thirty million North American men are affected and suffer with some form of erectile dysfunction (www.mensclinic.com).

By definition, erectile dysfunction, is "the inability to achieve or sustain an erection for satisfactory sexual activity, also known as impotence" (www.medicinenet.com).

Experts believe that there are many contributing factors to erectile dysfunction, including lifestyle choices such as smoking, being over-weight, and lack of exercise. Drugs such as blood pressure mediation, anti-depressants, tranquilizers and appetite suppressants also can contribute to erectile dysfunction. Hormonal abnormalities (low levels of testosterone) and psychological factors such as anxiety, stress, guilt and depression have also been recognized as contributing factors to creating erectile dysfunction. This topic of erectile dysfunction is not easy for men to discuss with either their health care professionals, or their partners. However, this condition is one that is related to an imbalanced endocrine system (stress, anxiety, depression) as well as an imbalanced reproductive system. With the average Canadian couple engaging in sexual intercourse seven times per month on average (www.edhelp.ca), the ability to perform sexually is important.

A survey of a cross-sectional sample of 3,921 Canadian men ages forty to eighty-eight years seen by primary care physicians reported that fifty per cent of Canadian men over forty years of age suffer with some degree of erectile dysfunction. (www.edhelp.ca).

Erectile dysfunction is very common and there are many different ways to improve this imbalance and the use of the superfood Maca on a consistent basis is most definitely a great option!

A double blind clinical trial with fifty Caucasian men affected with mild erectile dysfunction was conducted. The men were given a 2400mg dose of dry Maca extract per day in comparison to a placebo group. The study was conducted over a twelve week period and the data supported a small but significant improvement for general and sexual well being in adult patients with mild erectile dysfunction by supplementing with Maca. In this study, only the Maca treated patients experienced a significant improvement in physical and social performance. (www3.interscience.wiley.com).

Maca is known to naturally increase the levels of testosterone in men and that is a major factor in balancing the endocrine system and eliminating the symptoms of erectile dysfunction. In addition to being a hormone balancer, Maca also contains a high amount of amino acids, specifically arginine. Arginine is an amino acid that provides increased oxygen production and as a result promotes better circulation within the body and assists to promote better oxygen flow to the male reproductive system. This increase in oxygen enhances erections and sexual function. According to the Mayo Clinic, "Arginine changes into nitric oxide, which causes blood vessel relaxation (vasodilation)." "Early evidence suggests that arginine may help treat medical conditions that improve with vaso-dilation, such as chest pain, clogged arteries (called atherosclerosis), coronary artery disease, erectile dysfunction, heart failure, intermittent claudication/peripheral vascular disease and blood vessel swelling that causes headaches (vascular headaches)". (http://www.mayoclinic.com/health/l-arginine/NS_patient-arginine).

Maca not only increases testosterone and provides the popular hor-mone-enhancing benefits, but Maca also provides quality nutrients such as high potency amino acids that assist with improving sexual health among men of all ages.

Maca Protocol:

One teaspoon of **MacaPunch XP Platinum** liquid, four to six times daily or three capsules of Brad King's **Ultimate Maca Energy** four to six times daily.

Nutrition Tip:

Incorporate foods that are wholesome such as the foods listed in Appendix A- Introduction to a Whole Foods Lifestyle.

Include four to five servings daily (one serving is equivalent to ½ cup) of anti-oxidant rich foods. This includes raw vegetables such as broccoli, spinach, green beans, beets and includes fruits such as grapes, kiwi, blueberries, raspberries and strawberries. These types of food contain high levels of antioxidants, which will assist with increasing oxygen within the body. This is important as one of the health issues with erectile dysfunction is not enough oxygen is flowing to the male's reproductive organ.

In addition to my point above, decrease your intake of pro-inflammatory foods such as pork, beef, dairy, potatoes, tomatoes, eggplant and peppers. It is important that you consume foods that are going to improve oxygen flow in the body, not impair it.

Lifestyle Suggestions:

If you are a smoker, Quit! Smoking is one of the contributing factors to erectile dysfunction, not to mention heart disease and overall decrease in life span. Each cigarette reduces the oxygen going into the veins and arteries. If you are suffering with erectile dysfunction, it is very likely that your body is not getting enough oxygen and this is creating an imbalance in the reproductive system.

Male Fertility and Maca

We have already discussed in great detail fertility in women earlier in this book. It was once thought that if a couple was not able to conceive that it was the result of an imbalance within the female's system. However, with more sophisticated research, we now know that information is simply not true. Men can suffer with infertility issues as well. However, due to many years of research and with the option of alternative therapies, there is a safe and effective solution for men struggling with this issue. The solution is MACA!

Researcher Dr. Gustavo Gonzales conducted a trial with a sample of men twenty to forty years old to reveal the effect of gelatinized Maca on adult men. The men in the study were given Maca or a placebo to use consistently for one year and five months. At the end of this trial, there were many positive conclusions. Maca was found to be effective as an energizer and was also found to improve the male's state of mind, along with greatly increasing DHEA levels in the men using the gelatinized Maca. (According to the Mayo Clinic, "DHEA (dehydroepiandrosterone) is an endogenous hormone, made in the human body and secreted by the adrenal gland. DHEA serves as precursor to male and female sex hormones (androgens and estrogens)".(http://www.mayoclinic.com/health/dhea/NS_patient-dhea.)

Maca was also found to decrease anxiety in men within two weeks. A decrease in stress resulted in men appearing to handle stress more effectively. This trial reported that Maca improved the level of sexual desire in men, along with increasing the volume of sperm produced and sperm motility. This trial provided great support for the use of Maca within the male population for libido, energy, mental clarity and fertility. (Study-Effect of Lepidium Meyenii of Lepidium Peruvianum (Maca) administered in form of gelatinized tablets).

The issues which have been discussed in all sections of men's health (Andropause & Maca, Aphrodisiac Activity and Enhance Libido & Maca, Erectile Dysfunction & Maca, Male Fertility & Maca) are all related to the decrease in the production of testosterone in men. Unfortunately, many men suffer in silence with their imbalances because their symptoms are not as obvious and let's face it – men are not as forthcoming with their health concerns as women tend to be. Even though men are not as willing to share their health concerns, there is still a great solution to offer them when they are ready. MACA!

The use of Maca will provide men with an improvement in their sexual health, a noticeable increase in energy, self-confidence and general well-being.

Maca protocol:

One teaspoon of **MacaPunch XP Platinum** liquid six times daily, or three capsules of Brad King's **Ultimate Maca Energy** six times daily.

If you find that you begin reducing the dosage of Maca and your symptoms return, then increase the dose for an additional four weeks.

Try to reduce the dose after four weeks again. Everyone's bodies and hormones may require a slightly different dose, so be comfortable with adjusting your intake of Maca to provide balance to your system and eliminate your symptoms.

Nutrition Tip:

Along with balancing testosterone levels with Maca, improving the diet is also recommended. Incorporate a whole foods lifestyle, Refer to Appendix A for the Introduction to a Whole Foods Lifestyle.

Eliminate all white flour, artificial sugars, processed and packaged foods from your diet. It is important that when you are attempting to balance your body systems (nervous system and reproductive system) that you fuel your body with optimal nutrition.

Include four to five servings of lean protein at twenty to twenty-five grams per serving. (Refer to the appendix B with the list of quality protein sources). Protein intake is very important for men as they benefit from the amino acids that naturally occur in protein sources.

Increase your intake of fruits and vegetables. These foods contain high antioxidants and will assist with providing your body the nutrients it craves. Whether you are looking to improve energy or hormonal health, the body requires a rich source of vitamins and minerals that come from fresh fruits and vegetables.

Limit the amount of stimulants that you ingest, such as caffeine, alcohol, smoking and drugs. Following the suggested nutrition plan will assist you in improving your system overall and allow the Maca to work more efficiently.

Supporting your body with optimal nutrition and quality nutritional supplementation will allow you to have a balanced, healthy body, and you will feel optimal all the time!

Osteoporosis and Maca

Osteoporosis is a growing health concern in both males and females. Osteoporosis is a condition in which the bones in the body lose density and mass. The bones become brittle and porous. When the bones begin to develop this condition, they are more susceptible to fractures and breaks.

In Canada, one in four women over the age of fifty have osteoporosis and one in eight men over the age of fifty show signs of osteoporosis (www.onehealthlifestyle.com).

According to the 2004 Report of the Surgeon General on Bone Health and Osteoporosis, "One out of every fifty women over (the age of) fifty will have an osteoporosis-related fracture in their lifetime with risk of fracture increasing with age."

There are several risk factors related to osteoporosis. These risk factors include "broken bones after fifty years of age, thin or small frame, consumption of three or more alcoholic beverages per day, and smoking cigarettes" (www.reclast.com). Research supports that hormonal health can play a role in the degree of osteroporosis an individual suffers with or becomes susceptible to.

According the Mayo Clinic, hormones in both men and women can be a factor that affects an individual's bone density. In women, when the female sex hormone estrogen decreases production during menopause, bone density dramatically decreases. Typically, women suffer more bone loss in the first five years after menopause. Therefore, optimal levels of estrogen are required to assist with keeping bones strong. When a woman enters menopause and estrogen production begins to decrease, so does her bone density.

The same research reported that a decrease in the production of estrogen and testosterone in men can also cause decreasing bone mass.

Jorge Aguila Calderon, MD and Dean of the Faculty of Human Medicine at the National University of Federico Villareal in Lima, Peru, prescribes Maca for a wide variety of health conditions, including osteroporosis and the healing of bone fractures in the very elderly. Calderon says, "Maca has a lot of easily absorbable calcium in it, plus magnesium and a fair amount of silica, which we are finding very useful in treating decalcification of bones in children and adults"(Hilgan Enterprises Inc).

Additional hormonal risk factors for osteoporosis are the imbalance of the thyroid gland. According to the Mayo Clinic, too much thyroid hormone in an individual's body can cause bone loss. Too much thyroid hormone can occur as a result of two separate conditions. The first is hyperthyroidism, when the thyroid gland is overactive and producing a high amount of thyroid stimulating hormone. And with the second condition, the individual suffers from Hypothyroidism (where the thyroid gland is not producing enough thyroid stimulating hormone) and therefore, the individual is taking excess amounts of hormone medication or supplementation to treat the under-active thyroid. With both conditions, the body has an excess of thyroid- stimulating hormone and too much of this hormone can create bone loss.

Osteoporosis is a serious condition and it is very interesting to learn of the contributing factors that create the imbalance within our bodies. With hormonal imbalance being one of the factors related to the cause of this condition, it is great to know that Maca can assist in managing this imbalance and dealing with the root of the problem. If an individual is suffering from osteoporosis along with unbalanced hormones, Maca would be a great nutritional superfood to restore the balance within the individual's system. The use of Maca for osteoporosis would allow the body to increase the required hormones to maintain a healthy bone density in both men and women.

Research has indicated that bone mineral density in fact improved when higher dose of an ethanol extract of Maca was given to rats. The research indicated that Maca was effective in the prevention of estrogen deficient bone loss (Zhang, 2006, April 21 – Effect of ethanol extract of L M W Pub med).

Maca Protocol:
One teaspoon of **MacaPunch XP Platinum** liquid, three times daily or three capsules of Brad King's **Ultimate Maca Energy** three times daily.

Nutrition Tips:
In addition to supplementing with Maca to restore the hormonal balance and maintain bone density, attention to diet is also a crucial component.

To promote healthy bone density, focus your food choices on the foods listed in *Appendix A – Introduction to a Whole Foods Lifestyle.*

Incorporate three to four servings (serving size is equivalent to ½ cup) of greens (spinach, kale, romaine, swiss chard). Also be sure to include two to three servings of raw vegetables such as broccoli, cauliflower, green bean, and beets as they are antioxidant vegetables which will decrease any unwanted inflammation in the body.

Eliminate the following foods, as they are pro-inflammatory and will only prevent healthy bone density. The pro-inflammatory foods are; artificial sugars, dairy, tomatoes, potatoes, peppers, eggplants, pork, beef, caffeine and alcohol.

Eating a sufficient supply of calcium rich foods will also assist with improving bone density. Below is a list of great foods that provide a highly absorbable form of calcium.

Three to four servings per day would be ideal. (one serving is equivalent to ½ cup).

Salmon	Almonds	Fruit Yogourt
Shrimp	Brazil Nuts	Plain Yogourt
Sardines	Hazelnuts	Goat cheese
Perch	Peanuts	Grapefruit Juice
Mackerel	Sesame seeds	Orange Juice
Broccoli	Flaxseeds	Rice Milk- Ryza
Kale	Walnuts	Soy Milk
Orange		Almond Milk

You will notice the chart above listing calcium-rich foods does not contain dairy from cows. This was not a mistake. As a holistic nutritionist and from what I have witnessed in my practice, dairy from cows can be a very pro-inflammatory food. I find that if the body is already inflamed or has a high acid content, then dairy from cows creates more of a negative issue. As a result, I do not recommend dairy from a cow as part of a whole foods lifestyle.

Immune Booster, General Well Being and Maca

M aca is an incredible immune enhancer. This super food is loaded with vitamins such as Vitamin A, B, C, D, and E. As well, Maca naturally contains zinc, glucosinolates and plant sterols, which are potent antioxidants and are known as immune enhancers.

With this incredible nutrient profile, Maca can assist to build a healthy immune system and as a result, provide an improved sense of well-being.

Nutrition Tips for a healthy immune system:

Eat Fresh, Whole, Raw Foods: This means shopping on the outer aisles of the grocery store, where there is fresh fruits and vegetables (as well as fresh meat and whole grain bread). Fresh, raw fruits and vegetables will provide your body with quality nutrients that will naturally boost your energy and your immune system! The foods located in the middle aisles are high sugar, high fat, high salt foods and filled with an abundance of preservatives to provide a long shelf life.

Eat a Variety of Foods: Each food on your plate should be a different colour. Each different colour of fruit and vegetable represents different nutrients. Green vegetables such as dark leafy greens (kale, spinach) are high in the minerals iron, calcium, potassium and magnesium. Dark green vegetables are also rich in Vitamin C & E and many of the B vitamins. Orange fruits and vegetables are high in fibre, vitamin A, C and K. Therefore, incorporating a variety of colours in your meals will ensure you are getting an assortment of vitamins and minerals.

Consume high anti-oxidants foods: blueberries, cranberries, greens, broccoli, spinach, kale, asparagus, garlic, pumpkin, sweet peppers, mango and sweet potatoes.

Athletes and Maca

Maca is a great energy booster and provides incredible nutrients for stamina and endurance. Maca is a wonderful product for an athlete if they are looking to improve their energy without over-stimulating their body.

Maca is loaded with immune boosting vitamins, energy-producing amino acids and the ability to promote balanced hormonal function.

Any athlete who chooses to use Maca as an energy booster will be very pleased with the results. Maca will not over-stimulate the adrenal glands (stress glands) and create more stress in the athlete's body while training. In fact, the use of Maca strengthens the adrenals, which will then assist with stamina and endurance in their sport.

Often due to over-training, inadequate nutrition and not enough rest, an athlete can suffer with Adrenal Fatigue. By consuming an adaptogen such as Maca, this will provide energy and repair the adrenal glands at the same time. The athlete will experience a better quality of energy and a more consistent and sustained energy.

Research was conducted evaluating the vigor-inducing effects of Maca. The results of this research showed a "significant increase of energetic performance in oxygen consumption and also an increase of resistance on swimming time." (Vigor-Inducing Effect of Maca (Lepidium meyenii Walp), an Andean Hypocotyl, in Mice, Salas CA. Draft Paper.

Another study was conducted on the effects that Maca has on physical-energetic performance in humans. The results of this study reported a significant improvement in physical-energetic performance within individuals supplementing with Maca compared to the placebo group. In this particular study, an increase in distance range was noted and as a result, stamina was also noted as having improved in those individuals supplementing with Maca (Effect of Lepidium meyenni (Maca) on physical performance in humans. Gayoso O, Aguilar JL, Goyzueta I, Rojas P, Marcleo A, Timoteo O, Carvajal L. Draft Paper).

TESTIMONAL FROM EMMA, 32

I have used Brad King's **Ultimate Maca Energy capsules** *for the past two years. Overall, Brad King's* **Ultimate Maca Energy capsules** *have given me the instant energy and stamina to combat my fatigue and improve my overall endurance and strength while engaging in resistance weight training. I found that using Brad King's* **Ultimate Maca Energy capsules** *for three months straight and taking one month off was beneficial for my personal use. As a mom, I find that Brad King's* **Ultimate Maca Energy** capsules *have all the benefits to help promote mental focus and energy, and I would highly recommend anyone to try this wonderful FOOD!! You will feel energized!!!!*

Ultimate Maca Energy powder is a great product to use before a workout session or a game, as it will provide the body with an enhanced energy with the consumption of all the vitamins, minerals, protein and carbohydrate content naturally found in Brad King's **Ultimate Maca Energy powder**. I would also recommend that an athlete add this nutrient-rich superfood to their after work-out protein shake to assist with replenishing the worked muscles. The protein found in Maca will assist with muscle repair, and the naturally occurring magnesium and fatty acids will aid in relaxation of muscles and reduction in inflammation from training the body.

Maca Protocol:

One teaspoon of **MacaPunch XP Platinum** liquid twice daily or three capsules of Brad King's **Ultimate Maca Energy**, twice daily.

Nutrition Tip:

One heaping teaspoon of **Ultimate Maca Energy powder** into a smoothie or a protein shake. (Refer to the Appendix for smoothie recipes with Ultimate Maca Energy powder).

As an athlete, it is important to include high antioxidant foods such as raw fruits and vegetables to assist with the build-up of inflammation in the muscles from working them so intensely. As an athlete, I would recommend that you include three servings (one serving is equivalent to ½ cup) at each meal with a combination of raw fruit and vegetables.

Ideally, one serving of fruit, and two servings of vegetables in the recommended three servings per meal.

In addition, I would limit the intake of pro-inflammatory foods such as pork, beef, potatoes, tomatoes, eggplant, peppers, white sugar and dairy.

Include good quality Omega 3 fats in your diet as well to supply the muscles with the necessary anti-inflammatory nutrients.

The Brain and Maca

Maca not only improves the functioning of the physical body, but this incredible superfood also provides nutrients to the brain to assist with the mental aspect of our health.

In the nutritional profile, Maca contains twenty fatty acids including omega 3, 6 and 9, along with 18 out of the 22 amino acids.

Good quality fats improve mental functioning of the brain such as improved mental clarity, better concentration and focus, as well as an improved memory. An article in *Psychology Today* reported the following: "Omega-3s are known to be particularly crucial constituents of the outer membrane of brain cells. It is through the fat-rich cell membrane that all nerve signals must pass. All brain cell membranes continuously need to refresh themselves with a new supply of fatty acids. A growing amount of research suggests that the omega-3s are best suited for optimal brain function." (www.psychologytoday.com/articles/200310/what-is-good-brain-food.)

Many customers and clients who have used Maca report after a short time, they notice an improvement in their mental acuity and many have even reported that they "feel like a fog has been lifted." I find this aspect of Maca so interesting. Many of us are so busy throughout our day that we often could use a mental pick- me-up. And it is great to know that consuming this incredible superfood will give us the perk that is much needed without any negative side effects. In fact, we are improving the balance of our health by using the nutrient-rich supplement.

Maca also contains an abundance of amino acids, which is another important nutrient that is beneficial to the functioning of the brain. Amino acids, which are naturally found in protein (Refer to *Appendix*

B for a list of Quality protein sources) are a necessary part of every living cell in our bodies. *"Certain amino acids are required for the brain to receive and send messages."* (Balch, Phyllis A. *Prescription for Nutritional Healing*, 4th Edition, 2006, pg51). Regular consumption of foods and nutritional supplements that contain high levels of amino acids assist with improving our communication skills. These nutrients essentially provide our brain with power and allow us to understand and respond to everyday communication.

The correct balance of amino acids is also necessary to balance mood and brain activity. Amino acids provide the brain with the nutrients required to function at its best and feed the brain to assist in regulation of hormones.

TESTIMONIAL FROM NORM, 63

Discovering Lorrie as a holistic health practitioner has been a life-changing experience for me. Along with a better diet, exercise and a new bride, the product **MacaPunch XP Platinum** *has rejuvenated me. I will spare the details about the new bride part, but over-all I have had increased energy both physically and mentally.* **MacaPunch XP Platinum** *has definitely had a positive impact on my life-style. I endorse it without reservation.*

Maca Protocol:

One teaspoon of **MacaPunch XP Platinum** liquid, twice daily or three capsules of Brad King's **Ultimate Maca Energy** twice daily.

Nutrition Tip:

Include a diet of whole foods (Refer to *Appendix A – Introduction of a Whole Foods Lifestyle*).

Increase your consumption of omega 3 fats; includes foods such as salmon, sardine, cod, snapper, halibut, shrimp, flax seed oil or ground flax seeds, and walnuts.

And of course eliminate unhealthy fats such as fast food or processed foods. These foods create inflammation and are not beneficial to your health. Omega 3 fatty acids are anti-inflammatory and will assist with improving your overall health.

Conclusion:

I hope you have enjoyed the information within this book as much as I enjoyed sharing it with you. As you are now aware, Maca is one miraculous superfood. With incredible healing properties, this fabulous root vegetable is one of the most nutrient-rich foods in the world. Maca has the ability to improve so many aspects of an individual's health – both male and female – with no known side effects.

As my dear friend always says; "If you do not take the time to care for your health now, then you better make time to be sick later." So begin taking care of yourself today…one teaspoon of Maca at a time!

Thank you for joining me on this wonderful journey and be well!

Frequently Asked Questions

Can Maca be used with other hormone balancing medications or supplements?

Yes! Maca is a food put into supplement form. There are not any known side effects of Maca, therefore you can think of Maca as you would a yam or a turnip. If you can eat these foods with your medications and supplements, then Maca is fine, too! I always recommend that you take supplements and medication three hours away from one another simply to improve absorption of the ingredients in the medications and supplements.

If you are unsure, then I would recommend you contact a holistic health care practitioner that is familiar with the healing benefits of Maca!

Is Maca safe for Children to take?

Yes! Maca is safe for children as there are no known side effects of taking this superfood. I would recommend that you provide Maca to children in the form of the gelatinized powder and mixed in with food. (Refer to the recipes located in the Appendix section). In Peru, infants and children consume Maca in the form of food as part of a healthy wholesome diet.

Can I take Maca if I am Pregnant?

If you were using Maca before you became pregnant, then yes, you can continue your use of Maca throughout your pregnancy. Although there is not any research that supports Maca is harmful during pregnancy, I would not recommend that you begin a supplement regime with Maca if you are pregnant and were not using Maca prior to becoming pregnant. I would make this recommendation with any supplement. If you were not taking the supplement prior to pregnancy, I would not recommend you begin the supplement after you have conceived.

Can Maca be given to my pets?

You will be happy to hear that the native Peruvians fed Maca to their livestock to increase strength, fertility and stamina. This wonderful superfood was shared with everyone, even their animals. It has been noted that when Maca is given to domesticated animals, it has greatly enhanced their health. As Maca does with humans, it will increase fertility and build healthy and happy offspring in the animal kingdom.

Where can I purchase Maca?

The **MacaPunch** supplement line and Brad King's **Ultimate Maca Energy** are sold in quality health food stores all over Canada. Be sure to ask your local health food store for this amazing product.

The **MacaPunch** Supplement line and Brad King's **Ultimate Maca Energy** is exclusively distributed in Canada through Preferred Nutrition. This top-quality supplement company is committed to providing products, information and people that are dedicated to keeping the industry healthy, well informed and feeling good.

Visit Preferred Nutrition online at www.pno.ca

APPENDIX A

Introduction to a Whole Foods Lifestyle

The holistic approach to nutrition is strongly based on the use of whole foods.

A simple definition of whole foods is: consuming food in the natural state in which it was grown. This means that foods should be eaten as whole pieces of fruit, fresh vegetables and grains that are not processed but still contain all three parts of the grain, (germ, bran and endosperm).

A whole foods approach to nutrition is literally going back to the basics and eating pure, whole unprocessed foods.

VEGETABLES:

Vegetables provide many nutrients that supply the body with energy, life and continuous vitality. A diet high in a variety of vegetables will supply you with an assortment of vitamins, minerals, fibre, enzymes and nutrients the body requires to function at its best. Choosing different vegetables each time you purchase your produce will ensure that your body is getting all the nutrients that it needs to run optimally and to maintain optimal health.

Vegetables contain many vitamins that strengthen our immune system and provide us with the natural protection we need to fight against the chemicals and pollutants that are found in our air, water and foods.

Vegetables also contain many necessary minerals that build strong bones, teeth and assist in keeping our body in balance.

TIP: When grocery shopping buy three to five different vegetables each time. Keeping this rotation will allow you to try new foods, as well as maintain a great variety of nutrients in your diet with very little effort or inconvenience.

FRUITS:

Fruits provide the body with high levels of antioxidants and bioflavonoids that are beneficial in boosting the immune system, improving the endocrine system, as well as assisting in prevention of many diseases. Many fruits contain high fibre and promote a healthy intestinal system which keeps the bowel moving regularly. Fruit is easy to digest as fruit contains its own enzymes which assist with the break down of this food during digestion.

PROTEIN:

Obtaining adequate protein is essential for growth and development within the body. Protein provides the body with energy and assists in building and repairing muscle. As well, protein is involved in manufacturing hormones, enzymes and tissues within the entire body. Most of us do not eat enough quality protein on a daily basis.

The following are quality forms of protein and should be incorporated into your daily diet:

Chicken	Legumes-chickpeas
Salmon	Eggs
Tuna	Turkey
Mackerel	Nut Butters- almond, peanut, pumpkin
Trout	Lentils
Sardines	Tofu
Beans	Shrimp

Brad King's Ultimate Protein (High Alpha or ISO Whey)

** Limit red meat and pork consumption to one to two times per week and incorporate more of the above proteins.

GRAINS:

Eating the proper kinds of grains that are rich in vitamins and fibre is extremely important and often the most neglected. The grains that are most beneficial to one's health are those that include the WHOLE grain, meaning the bran, germ and the endosperm of the grain.

These three components make up the entire grain. Many of the grains that we eat (white bread) do not contain all three components (bran, germ and endosperm) and therefore, are lacking in very important nutrients.

The body cannot efficiently use the ingredients in a non-whole grain product such as white flour products and will often tell you this through symptoms such as gas, bloating, headache, fatigue and possibly allergies.

The following grains are whole grains and should be incorporated into your diet daily:

- Buckwheat
- Rye
- Millet
- Flax
- Quinoa
- Spelt
- Wild Rice
- Kamut
- Brown Rice
- Barley
- Oats

FATS:

We all need fats in our diets daily! However, the types of fats we choose is what is most important.

"Good Fats" also known as essentially fatty acids (EFA'S) are not only healthy for us but they assist in regulating the entire fat metabolism so the body can function more optimally.

Good fats will nourish and lubricate the skin, assist in optimal brain function, regulate the nervous system and even assist in weight loss.

When our body ingests good fats, our system recognizes it as an essential nutrient, breaking it down and sending it through the body to be used in various body systems.

Choosing quality fats from the following list daily will ensure that you are getting the right kinds of fat in your diet:

These fats can be heated and used in cooking as they can remain stable with heat:

- Olive Oil
- Coconut Oil
- Butter

The following oils must remain cold or at room temperature for your system to absorb the quality nutrients. If these oils are heated, it will denature the oil and no longer provide the beneficial effects of these quality fats.

- Grape Seed Oil
- Raw nuts & seeds
- Safflower Oil
- Tuna
- Sesame Oil
- Walnut Oil
- Salmon
- Pumpkin Oil
- Borage Oil
- Sunflower Oil
- Evening Primrose Oil
- Mackerel

WATER:

The human body is made up of two-thirds water. Water is absolutely essential to our daily diet. If we are not getting adequate amounts of pure water, then our cells suffer from dehydration. In addition, water assists in transporting nutrients and waste products in and out of our cells. Without properly hydrated cells, our body suffers and the toxins that are in the body cannot be flushed out.

Water is necessary for the function of all body systems, as well as for the utilization of water-soluble vitamins.

One to two litres of water daily will assist in providing the body with the necessary supply to function optimally.

APPENDIX B

Protein with each meal

Protein-rich foods are the building blocks for tissue growth and repair. Cells cannot be formed without protein in your diet. They are used to form muscles, connective tissues, skin, hair and nails. Protein is also used to make hormones, enzymes and immune compounds to keep you healthy.

Protein content of selected foods (Grams) *3oz (90g) size of a deck of cards

Beef, 3oz (90g)*	21-25	Lentils, cooked, 1 cup (250ml)	19
Chicken, 3oz (90g)	21	Soybeans, cooked, 1 cup (250ml)	30
Salmon, 3oz (90g)	25	Soy ground round, 1/3 cup (55g)	11
Sole, 3oz (90g)	17	Tofu firm 6cm x 4cm x 4cm piece (80g)	13
Tuna, canned, ½ cup (125ml)	30	Veggie burger (soy based) 1 patty	12-14
Egg white, large (1)	3	Almonds, ½ cup (125ml)	12
Egg, whole, large (1)	6	Soy protein powder, flavoured, 1 scoop (28g)	14-16
Cheese, cheddar, 1oz (30g)	10	Soy protein powder, plain 1 scoop (28g)	25
Milk, 1 cup (250ml)	8	Whey protein powder 1 scoop (28g)**	22-25
Soy milk, 1 cup (250ml)	9	Mixed nuts, ½ cup (125ml)	13
Yogourt, flavoured, ¾ cup (175ml)	8	Sunflower seeds, 1/3 cup (75ml)	8
Beans, baked, 1 cup (250ml)	13	Peanut butter, 2 tbsps (25ml)	9
Black beans, cooked, 1 cup (250ml)	16	Kidney beans, cooked, 1 cup	16

** Suggested protein powder is Brad King's Ultimate Protein (High Alpha or ISO Whey)

Nutritious and delicious recipes with the fabulous healing benefits of Maca!

The recipes below are easy to make, nutritious and have the wonderful **Ultimate Maca Energy powder** added to them. This is another great way to get Maca into your daily diet. Enjoy!

Chocolate Peanut Butter Smoothie

INGREDIENTS:

½ cup	of chocolate soy milk
2 tablespoons	of all natural peanut butter/almond butter
1 scoop	of vanilla or chocolate protein powder*
1	small banana
1 tablespoon	of Ultimate Maca Energy powder
2	ice cubes

* Suggested protein powder is Brad King's Ultimate Protein (High Alpha or ISO Whey)

INSTRUCTIONS:

Place all ingredients into the blender and blend until smooth

Individual serving

Pineapple Smoothie

INGREDIENTS:

½ cup	pineapple juice
6 tablespoons	of silken tofu or biobest plain yogourt
1	small banana
1 tablespoon	of flaxseed oil
1 tablespoon	of Ultimate Maca Energy powder
1 cup	of strawberries or blueberries

INSTRUCTIONS:

Place all ingredients into blender, blend until smooth.

Rice/Almond Milk Smoothie

INGREDIENTS:

1 cup	of Ryza Rice Milk/ PC organics Rice Milk or Almond Breeze Original
½ cup	of frozen blueberries
1	medium size banana
1 scoop	of vanilla whey protein powder*
1 tablespoon	greens powder supplement
1 heaping teaspoon	of Ultimate Maca Energy powder

* Suggested protein powder is Brad King's Ultimate Protein (High Alpha or ISO Whey)

INSTRUCTIONS:

Place all ingredients into a blender.

Strawberry-Banana Breakfast Muffins

INGREDIENTS:

4	egg whites
½ cup	unsweetened applesauce
½ cup	sucanat (evaporated cane juice)
1 ½ teaspoon	vanilla extract
2	large bananas (mashed) or 3 regular size
½ cup	light buckwheat flour
½ cup	brown rice flour
1 cup	rye flour
1 teaspoon	of baking soda
1 tablespoon	of ground cinnamon
1 tablespoon	of Ultimate Maca Energy powder
1 ½ cups	slice strawberries OR 2 cups of fresh blueberries

Option:

Add 2-3 scoops of quality protein powder.

INSTRUCTIONS:

1. Preheat oven at 365 F and lightly grease muffin tray with unsalted butter.
2. In a large bowl, whisk egg whites, applesauce, sucanat, vanilla and bananas.
3. In another bowl, mix flour, protein powder, baking soda, cinnamon and maca powder. Stir flour mixture into the banana mixture until entire mixture is moistened. Stir in strawberries.
4. Spoon batter into muffin cups half full. Bake for 15 minutes or until done. Let cool before removing from tray.

Whole Wheat Scones

INGREDIENTS:

3 cups	of whole wheat flour
2 tsp	baking powder
1 tsp	baking soda
1 tablespoon	of Ultimate Maca Energy powder
Sprinkle	of sea salt
1 cup	buttermilk
2 large	eggs
2 tbsp	of sucanat (evaporated cane juice)
4 oz	melted butter

INSTRUCTIONS:

1. Combine together the flour, baking powder, soda, maca powder and salt.
2. Combine buttermilk, eggs and sucanat. Stir well.
3. Add approximately 2/3 of the dry ingredients to the buttermilk mixture. Stir well.
4. Add melted butter and remaining flour. Mix well.
5. Scoop out approximately 1/3 of a cup and place on a lightly greased baking sheet for 15 minutes at 350 degrees.
6. With scones, you can use cookie cutters to make them completely round or you can take a small amount in your hand roll it together and give it a little twist before placing it onto the baking sheet.

Makes approximately 20 scones.

Options to spice up your scones:

- **Cheese and chive:** grate your favourite cheese and chop chives, then add to the mixture as your last step.
- **Cinnamon:** In a bowl pour ½ cup of sucanat and ¼ cup of cinnamon, then roll the scone into the bowl to coat the outside before placing onto the baking sheet.
- **Apricot & Gogi berry:** chop up the apricots and gogi berries and then add as the last step to the mixture before placing the scones onto the baking sheet.

Whole Grain Banana Pancakes

INGREDIENTS:

1 ¼ cup	of oats
1 ¼ cup	of almond milk
2	egg whites
1 tablespoon	of olive oil or coconut oil
1 cup	of whole wheat flour
1 teaspoon	of baking powder
1 tablespoon	of Ultimate Maca Energy powder
2	mashed bananas

OPTION/EXTRAS:

- Add ½ cup of any fruit of your choice
- Add chocolate chips or gogi berries or BOTH!!
- Add 1 scoop of vanilla protein powder

INSTRUCTIONS:

1. Combine oats, maca powder and almond milk, allow to sit for 5 minutes.
2. Add the, egg whites, oil, whole wheat flour and baking powder.
3. Once that is almost mixed, add the banana and extras.
4. Cook in a hot pan or on a hot griddle.

Serves 8

Banana Bread/Muffin

INGREDIENTS:

¾ cup	of sucanat (evaporated cane juice)
½ cup	of melted butter
3	banana mashed
2	eggs
1 ½ cups	of whole wheat flour
½ tsp	baking soda
½ tsp	salt
1 tablespoon	of Ultimate Maca Energy powder

INSTRUCTIONS:

1. Mix together the sucanat, whole wheat flour, baking soda, salt and maca powder.
2. In a separate bowl, mix together the mashed bananas, melted butter and eggs.

3. Add dry ingredients to wet ingredients, and mix lightly.
4. Fold in any extras (see extras below)
5. Grease a loaf pan and bake for 1 hour at 350 degrees.
6. If you would like to make muffins with this recipe, then grease a muffin pan with butter and bake for 25 minutes at 350 degrees.

EXTRAS:

To spice up your banana bread you can add:
- Chocolate chips
- Walnuts
- Pecans

Cucumber-Avocado Soup

This recipe is simple to make and is great as a chilled soup.

INGREDIENTS:

1	ripe avocado, cut in small chunks
2	cloves garlic, minced
1	shallot, minced
½	English cucumber, grated
1 cup (450ml)	kefir or goats milk yogourt
½ cup	sparkling water
1 tablespoon	lime juice
2 tablespoon	cold-pressed flax oil
1 teaspoon	of Ultimate Maca Energy Powder

Fresh herbs of our choice (parsley, dill, tarragon, thyme)

Pinch	ground nutmeg

Sea salt and freshly ground pepper to taste

INSTRUCTIONS:

1. In a large bowl, thoroughly combine all ingredients, making sure the cucumber is not too watery. Cover and refrigerate at least 1 hour before serving.

No Bake Protein Bars

INGREDIENTS:

2 cups	quick cooking oats
1 ½ cups	all natural peanut butter or almond butter
4 scoops	of chocolate, or vanilla, or chocolate peanut butter protein powder*
1 tablespoon	of ground flax seed
1 tablespoon	of Ultimate Maca Energy powder
½ cup water	

* Suggested protein powder is Brad King's Ultimate Protein (High Alpha or ISO Whey)

INSTRUCTIONS:

1. Knead all ingredients into a large bowl.

2. Line a square pan with wax paper. Spread dough into pan using a spatula.

OPTIONAL: Spread a thin layer of peanut butter on top.

3. Freeze for 30 minutes.

4. Remove from the freezer and cut into bars. Keep in fridge to stay fresh.

Serves 12-16

OPTIONS:

This recipe allows you to be very creative. Choosing different flavours of protein powders will keep this recipe interesting.

Granola Bars

INGREDIENTS:

2 cups	of oats
4 cups	of assorted raw nuts and seeds (cashews, almonds, sesame seeds, sunflower seeds, pecans)
½ cup	chopped dried fruit (dates, raisins, apricots, dried cranberries, goji berries)
½ cup	of sucanat (evaporated cane juice)
½ -3/4 cup	of honey
½ cup	butter
2 teaspoons	of cinnamon
1 tablespoon	of Ultimate Maca Energy powder

INSTRUCTIONS:

1. Lightly butter a cookie sheet (with butter- unsalted).
2. In a large bowl combine oats, maca powder, nuts, seeds and/or fruit.
3. In a saucepan, melt butter.
4. Add sweeteners, stirring until blended.
5. Stir this wet mixture into the dry mixture and combine thoroughly.
6. Press into prepared pan and bake at 325 F for 20-25 minutes until lightly browned.
7. Cool for 5 minutes and cut into squares or bars. Let cool completely before removing from pan.

Guacamole

INGREDIENTS:

2-3	ripe avocadoes
1/4	of a small red onion chopped finely
1-2 teaspoons	of freshly squeezed lemon (can add more)
1 pinch	of cayenne pepper (can add more)
1 teaspoon	of Ultimate Maca Energy powder

Sea salt and pepper to taste

INSTRUCTIONS:

1. Mash avocadoes all together
2. Add red onion and lemon juice
3. Add cayenne and maca powder
4. Mix all together

**Can add chopped tomatoes

Hummus

INGREDIENTS:

2 cups	of chickpeas (not canned)
2	medium garlic cloves
¼ cup	fresh lemon juice
¼ cup	tahini
¼ teaspoon	cumin
1 tablespoon	of Ultimate Maca Energy powder
½ teaspoon	sea salt

Reserve chick pea cooking liquid

INSTRUCTIONS:

1. Soak chickpeas overnight in LOTS of water.

2. Drain chickpeas and place into a large cooking pot. Add 6 cups of water to the cooking pot. Boil on high 30 minutes, or until the chickpeas are soft and not crunchy.

3. Place garlic, lemon juice and ½ cup of chickpeas with ¼ cup of cooking water in the blender and food processor. Blend until smooth.

4. Add remaining chickpeas, cumin, maca powder and sea salt. (add small amount of cooking water for desired consistency). Blend until smooth.

5. Transfer into a bowl and mix tahini by hand.

Quinoa Salad

INGREDIENTS:

1 cup	of quinoa, rinsed (brown rice/wild rice)
2 cups	pure water
½ cup	dried cranberries
¼ cup	chopped fresh parsley or cilantro
1 tablespoon	extra-virgin olive oil (cold pressed)
2 tablespoons	of flaxseed oil
2 tablespoons	of Ultimate Maca Energy powder
2 tablespoons	of lemon juice
2 cups	chopped celery
¼ cup	chopped pecans, lightly toasted (could also use pumpkin seeds)
1-2	gloves of garlic, chopped finely

Sea salt and pepper to taste

INSTRUCTIONS:

1. Quinoa MUST be rinsed well, otherwise it will have a bitter taste. In a bowl of water, grind the grain between your fingers to rinse thoroughly. This takes about 2 minutes. Discard the rinsing water.

2. In a small pot, bring water to boil. Add quinoa. Lower heat to minimum, cover pot and simmer for 20 minutes.

3. Meanwhile, in a large bowl, combine all other ingredients.

4. After quinoa has cooled, combine with other ingredients in large bowl. Let sit for about 1 hour.

Can be served at room temperature as a warm salad or as a main dish, simply add beans, lentils, fish or chicken.

Serves 5-6

Vegetable Stew

INGREDIENTS:

2 tablespoons	of olive oil
1	medium onion, chopped
1	leek, sliced and washed carefully to remove any sand
8 oz	of firm tofu, diced sized cubes
2 cups	of pure water (or more if desired)
2	medium carrots, halved and sliced diagonally
1-2	large yams, diced
10-15	mushrooms, quartered
1-2	large garlic, chopped fine
1-14 oz	of diced tomatoes
1-19 oz	black beans
½ cup	of freshly chopped parsley
1 tablespoon	each of thyme, basil, marjoram and oregano
2 tablespoons	of Bragg's Aminos

Sea salt and pepper to taste

INSTRUCTIONS:

1. Fry onion, leek and tofu cubes in olive oil on medium heat for 5-10 minutes, stirring frequently.
2. Add the rest of the ingredients, plus just enough water to cover by 2 cm and simmer for ½-1 hour until vegetables are tender. Season with sea salt, pepper, Braggs and additional herbs to taste.

Yogourt Cheesecake

INGREDIENTS:

32 oz	(1 quart) Biobest
1 ½ teaspoon	of vanilla
1/3 cup	maple syrup
3 cups	of crushed graham crackers
½ cup	melted butter
2 tablespoons	of sucanat (evaporated cane juice)

| 1 tablespoon | of Ultimate Maca Energy powder |
| 2-4 cups | berries or sliced fruit |

INSTRUCTIONS:

1. The night before you plan on serving the pie, prepare the yogourt;

- Line a colander or large sieve with overlapping coffee filters.
- Place the colander or sieve in a large bowl.
- Spoon in yogourt and cover with a plate.
- Refrigerate for at least 10 hours. (after 3-4 hours pour out the liquid collected in the bowl and return to the fridge.

As the water drains, the yogourt will become the consistency of the cream cheese.

Discard all liquid at the end of the 10 hours.

2. Mix in the vanilla, maca powder and maple syrup by stirring it into the yogourt.

TO PREPARE THE CRUST:

In an 8 or 9 inch pie pan, mix the graham cracker crumbs with the melted butter and sucanat. Stir well and press into the pie pan evenly. Spread the yogourt over the crust.

Top the cheese cake pie with seasonal fruit.

It tastes best if you let the cheese pie chill for at least 30 minutes once it is all put together.

Serves 6-8 people.

Oatmeal Chocolate Chip Cookies

INGREDIENTS:

2 1/3 cup	of quick cooking organic rolled oats (not instant)
1 ½ cups	of whole wheat pastry flour
¾ cup	of applesauce
2 teaspoons	of non-aluminum baking soda
½ teaspoon	of sea salt
¾ cup	of sucanat (evaporated cane juice)
1 tablespoon	of Ultimate Maca Energy powder
1	large egg
1 teaspoon	of vanilla

1 cup	of carob chip or dark chocolate chips/milk chocolate chips
½ cup	raw nuts (pecans, walnuts, chopped almonds, sunflower seeds)
½ cup	of raisins

OTHER OPTIONS:

| ½ cup | of dried cranberries instead of raisins |
| ½ cup | of white chocolate |

INSTRUCTIONS:

1. Preheat the oven to 180C/350 F
2. Combine oats, whole wheat flour, maca powder, baking soda and sea salt into a large bowl.
3. Use an electric mixer to cream applesauce and sucanat together until they are light and fluffy. Beat in egg and vanilla.
4. Stir wet mixture into flour mixture.
5. Add carob chips nuts and raisins. Mix well.
6. Spoon 1 ½ -2 inches apart onto lightly greased cookie sheet . (grease with butter)

Makes 24 small cookies

Banana Berry Delight

INGREDIENTS:

Chocolate Delight:

3	ripe organic bananas
1 tsp of	freshly squeezed lemon juice
6 ounces	of semisweet organic chocolate (70 per cent cocoa)
10 ounces	of silken tofu (for a more firm pudding use firm tofu)
1 tbsp	of honey
1 tablespoon	of Ultimate Maca Energy powder
¼ cup	of ripe berries

INSTRUCTIONS:

Place all the ingredients, except the berries in a food processor or blender. Add them one at a time and blend before each addition until the mixture is smooth and creamy. Transfer to a serving dish and stir in berries.

Chill before serving. *Serves 4-6*

Milk Chocolate Brownies

INGREDIENTS:

¾ cup	milk chocolate, or unsweetened chocolate
½ cup	soft unsalted butter (leave the butter sit out on the counter over night)
½ cup	unsweetened apple sauce
1 ½ cup	sucanat (evaporated cane juice)
5	eggs
1 ½	teaspoon vanilla extract
1 tablespoon	of Ultimate Maca Energy powder
1 cup	whole wheat flour (use ¾ cup for more fudge-like brownie)

INSTRUCTIONS:

1. Lightly grease a 9 x 13 baking pan with unsalted butter
2. Preheat oven to 350 F
3. In a double boiler melt chocolate (boil a pot of water and place a bowl on top, place chocolate in bowl on top). Slowly stir the chocolate. Let chocolate cool for 10 minutes.
4. Cream the butter, apple sauce, and sucanat into a medium sized glass bowl until light and fluffy
5. Crack eggs into a separate bowl and using a fork, whip them for 1 minute.
6. Add eggs (1/4 each time) to the butter, sucanat mixture, maca powder and beat with a hand beater after each ¼ egg has been added. Stir in vanilla.
7. Stir while adding the melted chocolate. Once all the chocolate is added beat well for 1 minute with hand beater
8. Stir in flour
9. Mix well enough just to mix all ingredients together (If you over- mix, the brownies will be tough and spongy)
10. Spread batter into the greased pan.
11. Bake for 15 minutes, then turn in the oven for the remaining 10 minutes. Insert a tooth pick or knife and be sure they are cooked all of the way through. (the toothpick or knife should come out clean if cooked all the way through)
12. Let cool for 10 minutes before serving.
13. Cut into 12-16 pieces

**** To spice up the brownies you can always add nuts, dried fruit, grated orange peel, banana, coffee, etc. Simply add these ingredients in Step 7 after you have blended the chocolate together.